CARING
FOR THE BURNED

CARING
FOR THE BURNED

LIFE AND DEATH
IN A HOSPITAL BURN CENTER

By

JAMES M. MANNON, Ph.D.

Associate Professor of Sociology
DePauw University
Greencastle, Indiana

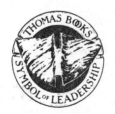

CHARLES C THOMAS • PUBLISHER
Springfield • Illinois • U.S.A.

Published and Distributed Throughout the World by
CHARLES C THOMAS • PUBLISHER
2600 South First Street
Springfield, Illinois 62717

© *1985 by* CHARLES C THOMAS • PUBLISHER

ISBN 0-398-05089-9

Library of Congress Catalog Card Number: 84-16294

With THOMAS BOOKS *careful attention is given to all details of manufacturing and design. It is the Publisher's desire to present books that are satisfactory as to their physical qualities and artistic possibilities and appropriate for their particular use.* THOMAS BOOKS *will be true to those laws of quality that assure a good name and good will.*

Printed in the United States of America
Q-R-3

Library of Congress Cataloging in Publication Data

Mannon, James M., 1942-
    Caring for the burned.

        Bibliography: p.
        Includes index.
        1. Burn care units — Social aspects. I. Title.
    [DNLM: 1. Burns — therapy. 2. Intensive Care Units.
    WO 704 M285c]
    RD96.4.M35 1985   362.1'9711   84-16294
    ISBN 0-398-05089-9

PREFACE

THIS book is the product of a two year participant-observer study of a hospital burn center in the Midwest. During that period, I spent many hours observing the daily interactions among patients and staff in an adult burn unit and one designed for children. My goal was to gain some insight into the social world of burn recovery, and to see that world, as best I could, from the viewpoint of the participants themselves. CARING FOR THE BURNED starts from the premise that certain problematic features of the burn care setting require participants to confront or cope with those problems, so that goals and objectives can be satisfied. As these problematic aspects of burn recovery are confronted and dealt with by participants, the basic social organization of the setting emerges. A hospital burn unit, like any setting, can be understood in terms of the social arrangements of norms, values, goals and interactions that comprise its social order. And, this is a social order that the participants create and shape in meeting the problems of the day.

CARING FOR THE BURNED is an ethnography and must be understood as such. I tried to be objective and neutral in making the observations, and I sought to be careful and accurate in generating the analysis. I did not begin with preconceived theories or analytic categories. As in much ethnographic work, I attempted to ground the analysis in the observational and interview data.

The reader should be aware that the conclusions and implications drawn in this book are mine alone, and are the product of observations made of a particular hospital setting and at a certain point in time. Social settings change, and it is possible, that in the time it has taken me to write this book, some of the procedures, philosophies and approaches to burn care described here may have been altered.

I have learned that burn units in general are open to exploring new ways to treat the criticaly burned, thus, approaches to treatment are evolving rather than static. The observations and analysis presented in CARING FOR THE BURNED should be seen in that light. It is my hope however, that the sociological insights into burn care made in this book, can contribute to more effective and humane approaches to burn treatment.

This study was made possible by a generous grant provided by the International Association of Fire Fighters Burn Foundation. Also, DePauw University awarded me a faculty research grant and a sabbatical leave to complete this research. I am grateful for the support DePauw has shown throughout this project.

I would like to pay tribute to all the surgeons, nurses, therapists, and others of the burn center staff, who allowed me complete access to their world, and total cooperation. Without their openness this book would have been impossible. Several surgeons and nurses were particularly helpful in permitting me to interview them. Out of these interviews came insights into the field of burn care, that I could not have obtained by observations alone. Because of assurances of anonymity, I cannot thank these persons by name, but they know who they are.

I am gratefuly also to the staff of several other burn centers in the United States, who allowed me brief, but, important access to their facilities. My visits to these centers provided me with perspective on the more general problems associated with burn recovery.

A number of friends and colleagues gave me ideas, help, and support at various points in this research, and I would especially like to thank: Charles Flynn, Deborah Bhattacharyya, Betsy Fife, Sarah Meadows, Ruth Sargent and Mary Knudson-Cooper.

My parents, James and Lucille, deserve a special mention for all the help and love they have shown me though the years. They made possible much of what has been good in my life. Also, my daughters, Susan and Sarah, like so many children do for their parents, have taught me more about myself than I deserve to know. This book is an expression of my gratitude to them.

Finally, I must acknowledge the many burn patients and their families who participated in this study. In spite of all that their ordeals were exacting from them, they never failed to be cooperative and open with me. To these patients, families, and all the members of the burn center staff, I dedicate this book.

"Everything that touches you shall burn you, and you will draw your hand away in pain, until you have withdrawn yourself from all things. Then you will be all alone."

The Seven Storey Mountain, Thomas Merton

"Either you love working with burns — our you hate it. There is no inbetween."

Burn-unit nurse, 1983

CONTENTS

CARING
FOR THE BURNED

Chapter One

INTRODUCTION

SHORTLY before noon, on a warm June day, Bobby Williams worked quietly putting the finishing touches on a new bumper he was welding to the rear of an automobile frame. Bobby was a college student during the school year, but in the summer he indulged in one of his true loves — working on cars. His job this summer, as a welder in Jake's Auto/Body gave him the chance to earn tuition money and also work at something he really enjoyed. The garage was very warm this morning, even with the large bay doors now wide open, but Bobby didn't mind, he liked the feel of the torch in his hands and savored its luminous glow as it forged steel on steel.

No one working in the garage, least of all Bobby, gave any notice to the several large, unfilled cans of paint thinner near the area where Bobby was working. And though the cans were virtually empty, their fumes, deadly and dangerous, began to drift slowly about the garage. Suddenly, without warning or provocation, these fumes found their way to the welding torch held firmly in Bobby's hands, and just as suddenly there was a small pop and explosion of flame that quickly ignited his clothes. Bobby was momentarily shocked, as if for a split second he didn't realize what had happened. But as the intense heat from the flames began to sear his flesh he knew he was on fire. Just as quickly his body's pain sensors now reacted and Bobby flew the first sensations of the most excruciating and almost indescribable pain he had ever known in his life.

Bobby ran shrieking from the garage, through the open bay door, frantically trying to tear the flame engulfed clothes from his body.

3

He searched desperately for some kind of blanket or tarpaulin to roll in or wrap around himself; and found none. He could not even find a patch of cool, thick grass upon which to throw himself. Realizing that the coarse gravel of the driveway would be his only bed he flung himself upon the stones and began to roll in agony. By now, and despite the intense heat and relentless pain, he had managed to rip off his shirt, but his work jeans had begun to melt into his legs, the large ornate belt buckle forming a molten mass that would not yield to Bobby's weak and painfully burned fingers.

One of Bobby's fellow workers, hearing his screams and seeing the flames had the presence of mind to telephone an ambulance. His message to the dispatcher was short and terse. "This is Jake's Auto/ Body and we've got a man on fire!"

The paramedic crew arrived shortly after the call was put in and when they rushed over to the spot where Bobby lay slowly wiggling, for now the flames were out, they could tell at once that he was terribly burned. No one in the crew had ever seen a body burned that badly and for a few brief moments they weren't sure where to begin. They knew he was alive, but barely. One of the paramedics began to cut away at the charred jeans while another prepared to check his air-way and vital signs. Bobby's face and throat had already begun to swell. The third member of the crew hurried back to the ambulance and instructed the dispatcher to call the regional burn center (sixty miles away) and tell them they would be bringing in a critical patient.

An hour's drive from where Bobby was now being carefully but swiftly loaded into an ambulance, Audry Young, the Head Nurse on the adult burn unit answered a phone call from the unit's medical director. "Audry, we just got a call from University City and they'll be bringing in a patient, a twenty-five year old male with a 90 percent burn. Their estimated time of arrival is about an hour." Audry took this message calmly, but in the back of her mind she knew that her nursing staff was already somewhat overworked, the burn unit rarely had an empty bed all spring and now Summer promised to be just as bad. Nevertheless, she realized to herself, "Well, this is what a burn unit is all about. But a 90 percenter. We'll have our hands full with him."

Audry walked down the hall of the burn unit where Vicky Casper was writing nursing notes in a patient's chart. Vicky had worked on the unit for less than a year but Audry had a lot of confidence in her. "Vicky we're getting new admisison. A twenty-five year old male with 90 percent burns. You want to get things ready? Dr. Nowicki is in surgery, but I'll page him. He had better be here for this one."

Vicky welcomed the chance to take charge of a new admission. This meant that a lot of the initial procedure details would be up to her and though she was still fairly new she felt she could get the job done. The thought of a 90 percent burn made her cringe just a little. Would he live, she wondered? Where would the surgeons get enough skin to graft all of that? She thought to herself, "If he does live, he'll be in here for a long time. He had better be strong!"

Susan, the physical therapist, was just walking out of the hydrotherapy room and Vicky stopped her. "Sue, we're getting a new admission in an hour. A 90 percenter. He's twenty-five years old." Sue look at her, "I'll help you get the tank ready if you want. We're finished for the morning." Vicky was pleased, "Thanks, Sue. I'll get a room ready and that will take awhile."

As Vicky walked to one of the equipment rooms, she rehearsed in her head some of the things she and the others on the burn team would need when the patient arrived. She knew that since he was a "big burn" she would have to get a heart monitor ready for his room, suction and plenty of IV fluids. She thought she better get four or five bags of fluid ready, a burn of that size will need at least that. Vicky stopped at the ward clerk's desk and asked her to call the emergency room and tell them the patient would be a "direct admit," meaning that when the ambulance arrived, the patient would be brought directly to the burn unit. They would handle all emergency and critical care functions right there in the unit.

Within a half hour most of the burn unit staff were aware that they were getting a big case and several of the nurses asked Vicky if they could help her get ready. She appreciated their offers, but since she still had twenty minutes she felt there was plenty of time to make the final arrangements. Near the end of the hour Vicky was working in the hydrotherapy room making certain she had plenty of blood tubes ready for they would be drawing a lot of blood cultures on this patient. He would be brought directly to the large spacious hydrotherapy room that could accomodate seven or eight people, members of the burn team who would begin their preliminary admission assessments and diagnostic work-ups. It is in this large room where every newly arrived patient is thoroughly examined for the extent and depth of the burn and accompanying injuries; and their medical histories are recorded.

As Vicky was busily checking her supply of blood tubes, Dr. Nowicki, a third year general surgery resident peeked his head through the door saying, "Vicky, they're on their way up. Is everythings all set?"

Vicky joined Dr. Nowicki in the doorway of the hydrotherapy room looking down the long corridor of the burn unit with nine rooms for patients on either side. Soon the double doors leading into the unit opened wide and two paramedics entered wheeling a stretcher began slowly moving up the hallway. Vicky was relieved to notice that they had started an IV line and were administering fluids. The form on the cart, draped in dry sheets, lay motionless, but his soft moaning became audible as they drew nearer to the hydrotherapy room. By now, several of the nurses and the physical therapist joined the procession and walked along the side of the cart.

Vicky could tell that Bobby was conscious, his eyes, though glazed over, had a pained and anxious look. She asked one of the paramedics as they wheeled him into the tank room, "What's his name?" "Bobby Williams," he answered. Vicky looked down into Bobby's swollen, reddened and sooted face, "Bobby, my name's Vicky and I'm going to be your nurse. You're in the burn unit at Memorial Hospital and the first thing we want to do is take a look at your burns."

The scene described above is based on an actual event that took place a year ago at the time of this writing. Only the names and a few of the features are changed to protect individual identities. Bobby was severely burned and he spent over three months as a patient in a hospital burn unit, where a burn care team comprised of surgeons, critical care nurses, physical and occupational therapists, social worker, and many consultants managed his recovery. Today, Bobby is mostly healed, and though he must periodically return to the hospital for reconstructive surgery, he is enrolled in college and will soon graduate.

According to recent estimates, in a single year nearly 300,000 persons in the United States will be hospitalized for burns, 20,000 of these will be treated in a hospital burn unit. Nearly 12,000 people will die as a result of burns, thousands more are scarred and disabled. Those who are treated in a burn unit will find their care managed by a group of people who think of themselves as a team, using a multi-skilled approach involving surgeons, nurses, therapists, social workers and various mental health experts. Much of the modern treatment of burns dates back to what was learned from treating victims of the 1942 Cocoanut Grove fire in Boston. The mass casualties resulting from that tragedy gave surgeons an opportunity to use new methods in burn wound recovery and gave impetus to a whole era of research and treatment of the critically burned that continues in several burn centers today.

While the team approach to burn care is characteristic of modern burn units, we have to date only a handful of studies and direct accounts about the workaday world of the men and women who elect to work with the acutely burned. This book seeks to fill some of that void, it is a sociological description and analysis of medical work in a hospital burn unit.

My focus in what is to follow, is partly on burned patients and their families, but mostly on the medical staff and their work since much less is known and written about them. In the most general sense, I tried to get an understanding of what it is like to work with the critically burned and to understand this from the pespective of several sets of participants, since not all participants or levels of staff will see it exactly alike. For example, burn surgeons face different uncertainties and demands than critical care nurses. But in a more specific sense, this study tries to get a feel for the social life of a burn unit that is to varying degrees shared by all. Medical work on the acutely burned can be exceedingly technical, complex, and sophisticated, yet sociologically we know that even this kind of work is always carried out within a social framework of values, norms, beliefs and interactions. That is to say, medical routines, procedures and judgments are never conducted in a vacuum or exclusively in those terms; they are always set within a social context, they have a social dimension. Thus, I'm offering an insight here into the medical world of burn care, the medical routines and procedures enacted upon the critically burned, but described and analyzed as essentially social behaviors that are guided, prompted and constrained by the various values, beliefs and norms of those who do this work.

Material for this book was gathered by direct observation and interviewing over a two year period. In all, over 600 hours were spent observing the daily routines in two hospital burn units including: surgery, doctor's rounds, dressing changes, hydrotherapy tankings, nursing reports, etc. I was given permission to conduct this study by the medical directors of an adult burn unit and a children's unit and they in turn secured the approval of their Department superior. The burn units described here were located in two large hospitals, one public and one private, both affiliated with the same medical school. Thus each of the burn units carried out a variety of teaching functions. Both hospitals were situated in the midst of a large medical school and hospital complex in the heart of a heavily populated midwestern city. The private hospital was a noted children's hospital and thus housed the children's burn unit, while the public hospital was general and provided the adult unit. Though the burn units were contained in separate hospitals, both were under the ultimate medical supervision of the same medical school teaching department (Plastic Surgery) and shared the same surgery residents. The adult and children's units were conceived as a regional burn center and treated the majority of the critically burned in the state.

The children's unit was a seven bed ward treating an average of about 60 acutely burned children per year. The adult unit contained nine beds and treated 115 burned adults in 1982. Each of the units was staffed by surgical residents, supervised by a medical director who was a staff surgeon; critical care nurses, physical and occupational therapists, a social worker, chaplain and a variety of consulting departments. While the staffing structure of the two burn units was similar, there were differences with respect to how certain routines were carried out and these issues will be described during the course of the book.

As in many participant observer studies of medical settings my initial interests and foci were rather broad and general as I explored the problematic aspects of working with the burned. Over time though my focus narrowed as I became sensitive to the features of the setting that seemed to undergird and in a sense organize muchof the work that was done. These features will be addressed in considerable detail in later chapters, but the reader will have a better grasp of what is to follow if I described them briefly here.

Trajectories

During the fieldwork phase of this study it became evident to me that the surgeons, nurses and therapists all had in common the need to create a kind of trajectory for their patients. These trajectories, or expected stages of recovery or dying, made their work more predictable and manageable. The concept of trajectory was introduced initially some years ago by Glaser and Strauss in their now classic studies of hospital dying and later refined in their investigation of pain management. The reader is asked to consult the bibliography in the appendix for the full citations of these works. As the recovery of burned patients involved a lengthy, arduous, painful and often complicated set of medical interventions and procedures, the burn unit staffs defined various recovery and dying trajectories for their patients. These trajectories took the form of expected phases or stages of death or recovery, that marked the progression of a patient to some end-state that included healing and recovery or dying and death. Burn care professionals established these trajectories because it gave them a set of explanations of what they expected to happen to burned patients and thus gave these staffs a framework for organizing their work and coming to terms with events that followed.

While creating dying and recovery trajectories was a way of organizing work and explaining what would happen to patients, I hope to show in subsequent chapters that these trajectories were not always easily arrived at, maintained or even agreed upon by all levels of staff. That is to say, the study of burn units with their emphasis on an interdisciplinary team approach gives us a unique opportunity to describe and analyze how these trajectories could become sources of disagreements and conflict among various members of the team.

Control

The second feature that began to capture my attention in the course of this research was the attempts on the part of burn unit staffs to gain greater control over their work situations. Because the burned patient was highly dependent on the staff (especially nurses and therapists), in that they were traumatized, physically immobilized, in great pain and psychologically anxious, staff needed to control the recovery situation in such a way to insure that routine procedures and activities went smoothly and the general working order was maintained. This included maintenance of the sentimental order, referring to the values and attitudes permeating much of the work carried out.

Within this general problem of gaining and maintaining control three distinct but interrelated problems also emerged. I'm calling the first of these independency/dependency and will attempt to describe this in terms of their basic tension. In the world of burn care, patients themselves were expected by staff to do as much as they could to aid in their own recovery. In a word, they were expeted to become "independent" - as fully and as soon as possible. This included being independent in activities of daily living; e.g. feeding themselves, brushing their teeth, walking to the bathroom, etc., as well as other independencies such as doing the physical exercise activities without being told or reminded to do so. Yet, because of the nature of a severe burn injury few patients were fully independent until the very final days of their hospital stay. Thus, there was always then an underlying tension with which the burn staff had to cope and come to terms between their needs to see patients become independent and self-reliant and the inescapable realities of burn trauma that produced a considerable degree of forced dependency. In looking at how burn unit staffs attempted to resolve this dilemma we have an opportunity to increase our understanding of the dynamics involved in all hospital rehabilitation programs.

The second problem that emerged under the general rubric of control had to do with the larger problem of patient compliance. As will be discussed more fully in a later chapter, burn patients were expected to "pick up thy bed and walk." The multitude of recovery activities for patients was often referred to by nurses and surgeons as "The Program," and patients were expected to embrace the program, see it as their own, and comply with it. In practical terms, burn patients were expected to maintain a certain level of calorie in-take each day, faithfully engage in their prescribed physical exercises, and wear their contracture splints and pressure garments to prevent scar formation. All of these requirements were very uncomfortable, painful, and trying ordeals for patients, but they constituted "The Program" and according to staff logic the only method whereby patients could recover from their disability and prepare to go home. Compliance then in the burn unit had to do with the various and sundry ways that staff created to get patients hooked into the program. Such activity became an important feature in staff's ability to control the recovery of burned patients.

Finally, the control of work on a hospital burn unit was problematic in other ways related to the interdisciplinary team approach. For no matter how each level of staff might have wanted to define their situations in ways that would make their work go more smoothly and routinely, as members of an interdisciplinary team they found their work activities inextricably linked with and dependent on the work of others. As an example, while the nursing staff might try to control the pain responses and behaviors of patients, if the surgeons failed or refused to give orders for certain pain medications there was little nurses could do other than to cajole, berate or persuade patients to respond differently; or to confront the surgeons directly in asking for a change in orders. Both roads were often taken by nurses not always successfully, and as we examine the work life in a hospital burn unit we can get a better understanding of the problems inherent in the multi-skilled approach to burn care specifically, and patient rehabilitation in general.

Engagement

The last of the three problematic features in caring for the burned was limited mainly to the work of nurses and therapists and it had to do with the ways nursing and therapy staff engaged burn patients in a kind of social and emotional bond during the course of treatment. In helping burn patients recover, nurses and therapists often developed strong emotional ties with patients. These ties were the product of a rapid upgrading of relationships to form intimate and mutual bonds of trust, but which were subject to abrupt endings when patients left the unit. Within the first few days of a patients entering the hospital, nurses and therapists engaged them on a first name basis and learned much about their biographical and family circumstances. In a sense, the nurses gave the patients an identity on the unit, and as the adult ward had very restrictive hours for family visiting, nurses quickly became the significant others for patients, and, at times, almost their surrogate families. Patients began to look toward the nursing and therapy staffs for self-approval, acceptance and social support. For patients who were facing many uncertainties in their recovery, e.g. the extent of scarring and disfiguration and functional loss of movement, the nurses and therapists became the one constant in their lives while in the burn unit. Within a context of sociability and shared trust, nurses and therapists were there for patients; to change their dressings, administer pain medication, rearrange their pillows, etc.; and patients came to rely on that constancy of response.

Nurses and therapists tended to use these strong interpersonal ties and dependencies to evoke a greater measure of patient compliance. For example, to the extent that patients looked to the nurses for approval and support, nurses were free to with-hold their approval when patients acted in ways considered inappropriate. Thus patients were often drawn into the recovery/rehabilitation program with its broad range of expected patient behaviors by the appeal of intimate interpersonal bonds with nurses who traded some measure of psychological engagement for greater patient compliance. When we look at this process in greater detail in Chapter Five, we will examine the several negative consequences of this process for nursing morale and patient recovery. For now it is enough to mention that this engagement process was fraught with difficulties in the cases of dying patients with whom nurses and therapists became emotionally committed as well as in the cases of those patients who frustrated themselves and nurses alike when they never quite lived up to the demands of the rehabilitation program.

This book is based almost exclusively on the 600 hours of direct observation of two hospital burn units. In addition, I conducted a number of in-depth and structured interviews with nurses, physical therapists, and surgeons. Not all burn units in the United States are structured alike and procedures such as surgical methods, wound care techniques and isolation policies will vary somewhat among different hospitals. In trying to ascertain some of the common problems facing all those who work with the burned, I made one and two day visits to several burn centers in the United States, including at least two of the most renowned programs with international reputations in burn care. As I toured facilities there and talked with various members of the burn unit staffs, I sought to get a feel for those commonalities. As a result, I'm confident in arguing that while

American burn units vary in several procedural routines and therapeutic philosophies, there are enough ways in which they are similar that analyis of a single burn center should yield important insights in understanding how the critically burned are cared for.

In this research I took the role of known observer, presenting myself as a sociologist interested in the daily life and routines on a burn unit. With this role, I was free to roam where and when I pleased on both the adult and children's wards. I often attached myself to a nurse or physical therapist and followed them as they did their work with patients; asking questions when appropriate and helping out if requested. For several weeks, I accompanied the surgery residents on their daily routines, meeting them at 7:00 a.m. when they made morning rounds in the burn unit and then going into surgery with them to observe surgical debridement, skin grafting and some reconstructive procedures.

On many occasions I stationed mysef in a single locale to observe all that transpired there in a period of several hours. The hydrotherapy room where patients are taken each day to have their dressings changed and wounds cleaned, is a very busy place each morning, and I would spend an entire morning at the side of the large Hubbard tank observing as nurses and therapists tended to a series of patients. The T.V. lounge was a favorite spot for ambulatory adult patients, and I often joined them in their conversations, watched T.V. with them and participated in the video games. I was even more active on the children's unit, helping to feed the children at meal times, and reading stories and playing games with those children who were well enough and old enough to appreciate the company.

Both units held weekly team conferences when all members of the burn care team would meet to discuss the progress and recovery of each patient, and I attended virtually all these meetings during a period of two summers. Monday morning grand rounds in which the medical directors and all other levels of staff would visit each patient's room to examine wounds and make surgical decisions, would find me bringing up the rear of the procession and being the last body sqeezed into the already crowded room.

As the study progressed and the nursing staff became more accustomed to my continued presence, I spent time in the nurses lounge sharing lunch and dinners with them and listening to their discussions of the day events on the unit. The nurses on the children's unit enjoyed cards and cross-word puzzles in their few free moments and eventually I was asked to join in, though my ability at cross-word puzzles was more greatly appreciated than my prowess at cards.

I tried to gain rapport by helping out in various ways to show that I was not adverse to getting involved. I ran errands to supply rooms, help lift patients on and off carts, delivered lunch and dinner trays for patients, took phone messages and was often an extra hand on dressing changes. On the children's unit I proved especially adept at rocking children to sleep during nap time, an ability that endeared me to the nurses. All the acts, small but not necessarily insignificant helped me gain some level of trust and acceptance from the staff. Such acceptance is not always total. In medical settings in general and burn units in particular there is always suspicion of strangers and a few of the staff never seemed comfortable having me around and maintained their distance from me. Most of the staff, however, appeared willing to have me around, some found me helpful and others fully accepted me as part of the team, if not medically astute, at least as enjoyable company and a good listener.

Like all observers, I was continually aware of the problems of over-rapport and identifying too strongly with the definition of reality of one set of participants. I sought to get as close to the burn unit staffs as possible, but not so close at to lose my objectivity and detachment. I was there as an observer; to objectivity describe, analyze and understand the work that went on, not to approve, judge or condemn it. No one set of participant's views was regarded as the "truth" and as a sociologist I did not have to share the interpretations of reality of the staff and patients, I had only to discover them and see where they fit within the frabric of the setting. How well I maintained my own detachment and objectivity and avoided seduction is for the reader to decide.

This book is written without the use of footnotes and references to scholarly works. I have done this to make the book more readable and engaging for the non-professional. My debt to other scholars in this research is considerable andI invite the reader to examine the appendix for a complete bibliography of the references that aided me enormously.

Also it should be noted that all names of persons, cities and hospitals are changed to protect identities. However, all the people described here are real and all the events described are based on actual happenings.

Chapter Two

THE SETTING

SHERI and Maureen, two nurses on the adult burn unit, were working quietly in room 208, word had been received about fifteen minutes earlier that a new patient would be arriving in about a half hour. As Sheri finished making the bed she asked Maureen, "I didn't hear anything about this patient, did you Maureen?" Without looking up from the chart in which she was writing, Maureen responded, "Someone said she's burned about 50 percent with face and neck involvement. But you know how that is . . . it might not be that bad. I guess she's in her forties and was using gasoline to clean some clothes or something. That's really all I know. They should be here around two o'clock." Sheri now turned her attention to checking the leads on the heart monitor as this would be the room they would give to the new patient. The room was neat, clean and orderly with fresh sheets on the bed. As Maureen walked out of the room she said over her shoulder, "I'm going to the tank room to make sure Art knows we've got a new patient. He'll want to get the tank ready to go."

Forty minutes later as Sheri and Maureen were walking down the hall toward the nursing station the double-doors at the entrance to the burn unit slowly opened and a paramedic with a yellow isolated gown over his uniform walked tentatively up the hall and stopped at the nurses station. Maureen asked, "Can we help you?" He answered, "Are you ready for Inez Nelson? We've got her right here at the door." Maureen told him, "Bring her on in but make sure everyone has gowns on."

16

Inez laid quietly on the stretcher as several ambulance staff wheeled her cart through the doors and then slowly down the hall where Sheri motioned them in the direction of the tank room. One of the paramedics nonchalantly held an IV bag of fluid up in the air a few feet over Inez's head.

When they had pushed the cart through the doors of the tank room, Maureen directed them to steer up next to another cart that was placed next to several large cabinets of medicines, supplies and packages of dressings. Sheri and Maureen were dressed as usual in their dark green surgical scrub suits that were preferred by all nurses in the burn unit. Since they would soon be looking at Inez's open burn wounds they wore disposable masks and hair nets. Sheri said to the paramedics, "We want to get her on our cart here, so let's lift her by this bottom sheet here. Watch out for the Foley bag."

Without too much effort Inez was gently and quickly laid onto the burn unit cart. Throughout all of this she hadn't spoken a word only an occasional soft but audible deep groan could be heard from her. Sheri looked down at Inez's face, which was swollen and puffy, and told her, "I'm Sheri and this is Maureen. We're gong to check you over for a few minutes to see how you are doing, O.K.? We'll start with your vital signs and then we'll draw some of your blood for tests. Your name is Inez — right?" Inez whispered, "Yes." "O.K. Inez, you just relax and we'll try not to hurt you," Sheri said. Sheri moved to the middle of the cart and began undraping the sheets that covered Inez's body, and as she did so Inez began to shiver as she was naked underneath. Maureen directed one of the paramedics, "There's a switch on the wall there for the heat lamps. Would you flip it on please? You'll feel warmer in a minute Inez, now I'm going to start drawing some blood and you'll feel a needle prick here. Just relax."

Inez was burned mostly on her arms, legs, back and neck. Much of the burn had already begun to blister and her legs and arms were crisscrossed with large wet blisters. Some of the skin on her left arm was burned reddish dark and dry and was splitting and peeling.

Inez had a nasogastric tube down her nose and Sheri began attaching one end of it to a suction device on the wall. This tube drains the contents of the stomach to prevent patients from vomiting and choking. As Sheri adjusted the suction tube she said to Inez, "Your face is swelling up Inez and your eyes may swell shut for a day or two. But don't worry about it, the swelling will eventually go down. Are you having any pain?" Inez answered quietly, "My arms hurt so bad." Sheri looked in the direction of one of the paramedics, "Did you give her anything for pain?" The one standing nearest to her responded. "We gave her eight of Demerol about two hours ago." Sheri and Maureen looked at each other and Sheri said, "Demerol? I think she better have some morphine." Inez winced and groaned out loud as Maureen inserted a large needle into her groin area to draw blood from one of the large veins there. Maureen heard Inez, but without looking up said, "I know that hurts, but we need this for tests. You're being real good Inez."

Bob and Joyce, two of the new medical students on the burn unit, had just made their way into the room and as Bob adjusted his mask he questioned Inez, "Are you allergic to any medicines?" "No," she moaned. "Have you had any surgeries?" Inez had difficulty speaking, but she managed, "I had a hysterectomy about five years ago." Bob asked her, "Do you remember what it was for?" "No . . . I can't remember now." Bob moved to the head of the cart and peered down at Inez's face. "That's O.K., just try to relax. Inez, we're going to have to put a new IV line up by your collar bone because your arms are burned and we can't use them. O.K.? I'll give you some numbing medicine so it won't hurt."

Bob searched the shelves for some sterile gloves and asked Sheri to get him a large bore catheter. Sheri aksed him, "Do you want a sixteen?" "That's all right, but a fourteen will probably do."

Inez called out feebly, "Has anyone told my husband?" One of the paramedics answered from across the room, "Inez we're getting ready to head back to Jackson and we'll try to find your husband for you."

By now Maureen had finished drawing the several blood samples and said to Bob, "I think she could use some morphine if that's O.K. with you." Bob answered, "Sure, why don't you give her four milligrams . . . she's not very big." Maureen looked at him, "four milligrams?" Bob straightened up and returned the stare, "Oh . . . I suppose you want ten? Well . . . O.K." Maureen peered down at Inez, "We're going to give you something for your pain and this will help you. You'll feel a lot better in a few minutes Hon."

On the other side of the large curtain that separated the area where Inez lay, Art, the physical therapy assistant was finished filling the large Hydrotherapy tank, called a Hubbard tank, with warm water and added disinfectant solution to it. It gave the water a foamy texture and yellow/brown coloration. Art knew that within a few minutes, Sheri, Maureen, and Sue, the physical therapist, would be putting Inez into the tank to clean her burn wounds, remove some of the already dead tissues and make their first judgements as to the depth and extent of her burns. Art propped himself up on the stool near the tank ready to help them with Inez, he predicted they would be needing the tank as soon as the medical student got that IV started.

All adult burn patients like Inez started their journey into the world of burn care by passing through those double entrance doors into the burn unit. They came in flat on their backs on a stretcher/cart and those who lived to recover usually walked out those same double doors to return to their community and families. For some, the recovery took only a few weeks, for others, several months would pass before they turned their backs on the burn unit. For all of them, it was an experience they would not soon forget. The reminders would always be there in the form of scars, disfigurations, stiffened joints and a myriad of physical and emotional aches and pains that never seemed to go entirely away. But part of those memories for patients will include the burn unit staff; surgeons, nurses and therapists who in various ways affected their lives rather profoundly.

To understand the social experiences of burned patients and the medical and nursing staffs charged with their care, we must start with the burn care setting, for it is this physical and temporal environment of the burn unit that shapes and molds the values and beliefs that permeate the care of the burned. Before we examine the setting and its participants more closely, however, it is necessary and helpful to make a brief excursion into the nature of burn injuries and their medical management.

Burns are the third leading cause of accidental death in the United States and the leading cause of death for children age 5 or younger. Among burned adults, occurances of drug abuse, alcoholism and emotional problems are higher than would be expected by chance. At least one study of burn cases reported that some 70 percent of those burned were victims of their own actions such as children playing with matches. Most burn injuries are caused by flames with scalds being the second leading cause.

Regardless of the cause of burn injury, all victims suffer loss of skin integrity. As the largest organ of the body, the skin has a number of important functions including protecting the body from infection by keeping out bacteria, preventing the loss of body fluids and controlling body temperature through evaporation of water from the sweat glands. Additionally, there are cultural values surrounding the skin's cosmetic appearance, especially the layers of skin on the face, neck, hands and arms.

The severity of a burn injury has to do with the size and depth of the burn. First degree burns (superficial) involve only the very top or epidermal layers of skin and usually heal in 5 to 10 days. Normally they would not require hospitalization. Second degree burns, sometimes referred to as partial thickness, extend into the dermis or deeper skin layers. They are very painful, and are usually moist, pale and frequently form large blisters. A deep partial thickness can take up to two months to heal. A full thickness burn injury, or third degree, involves the destruction of the entire dermis, sometimes including nerves, tendons and muscles. Here, nerve endings are destroyed and the wound is painless and insensitive.

The risk of medical complications from a burn injury is directly related to the total body surface area involved. Accordingly, the American Burn Association considers a severely burned patient as anyone with partial or full thickness burns over 20 percent or more of the body. For children, the percentage criterion is much smaller.

One of the problems surgeons and nurses face in evaluating the severity of a burn injury is that occasionally second degree burns can convert to third degree. If the patient is in poor physical condition with a number of chronic and serious illnesses aside from the burn injury, this conversion is more likely and adds to the clinical uncertainty in assessing severity of the burn.

The clinical treatment of burn injuries is thought to fall within three phases of patient care and are termed emergent, acute, and rehabilitative. The emergent phase immediately follows the burn injury in which the patient is in a state of physiological shock. There is a raid loss of fluid volume which is predictable and proportional to the size of the patient and extent of body surface area burned. This loss of fluids is very critical for patients and if fluids are not immediately replaced, the patient can suffer hypovolemic shock and die.

In the emergent phase, the burned patient is treated as any critical patient; surgeons work to maintain adequate respiratory and cardiovascular functions, maintain fluid balance and replace blood loss. In addition, a nasogastric tube will be placed into the patient's stomach for suction; a foley catheter inserted to maintain and measure urine output; and basic blood gases and serum chemistries will be obtained. The emergent phase can last anywhere from a few days to several weeks in the most critical cases.

The acute phase follows and it is a period of several weeks, depending on the time required to resurface those areas that had full-thickness skin loss. Surgeons are faced with deciding between two approaches to managing patients at this point; they must decide to resurface wounds using the conservative approach or taking the option referred to as immediate excision.

In the conservative method, surgeons wait for the eschar, which is the dead burned skin tissue, to separate from the healing granulation tissue beneath the wound. When this separation occurs and in the absence of wound infection, the granulation bed is thought to be ready to receive a skin graft. The surgeon will then take a layer of healthy skin from an unburned portion of the patient's body (called a donor site) and place it on the granulation bed. This is referred to as a skin graft and if it "takes," that is to say, the blood supply from the granulation bed permeates the graft, the patient's burned skin has thus been replaced and the wound is now closed and should heal.

The conservative method takes up to three or four weeks duration and is a somewhat complicated process. Prior to skin grafting, nurses and therapists must change a patient's wound dressings two or three times per day and also immerse the patient daily in the hydrotherapy tank. (In the case of smaller surface wounds, a shower is used.) Nurses encourage the eschar separation through a process known as debridement in which the dead tissue is removed by scissors and tweezers while the patient is immersed in the tank or during the dressing change. During this three to four week process, great care must be taken to prevent the infection of the burn wound. This is accomplished through the application of topical antimicrobial creams to the surface of the burn wounds.

The second option available to surgeons and one that appears with increasing frequency in American burn centers is known as aggressive debridement or early excision. In this approach, surgeons avoid waiting three or four weeks for the eschar to separate and opt to take a patient to surgery within a few days post-burn and surgically remove the eschar (excision) and close the wound surface with a graft of either the patient's own skin or pig or cadaver skin. Pig and cadaver skin are used as temporary substitutes when a patient is infected and surgeons fear that a graft of the patient's own skin will not "take," or when a patient lacks a sufficient amount of unburned skin from which to take a donor. Early excision is thought to lessen the time a patient must remain in the hospital and to save the patient many hours of painful debridement. However, burns greater than 15 to 20 percent total body surface area are difficult to excise in a single operation. Also, a patient might have a number of serious medical complications in conjunction with the burn injury and this could make surgeons reluctant to operate so soon after the burn and thus they might opt for the conservative approach.

During the emergent phase, the patient is much more aware of her/his surroundings and the many demands now being made to participate in her/his own recovery. Patients face the daily trip to the hydrotherapy tank for debridement; their painful dressing changes; fears of impending surgeries and the uncomfortable and painful program of physical exercise. It is within the emergent period that the nursing and therapy staffs are most concerned about the patient's morale and willingness to comply with all the demands associated with their recovery.

The last phase, rehabilitative, involves the process of getting the patient prepared to return home. Most burn patients have long convalescences after hospital discharge before they are ready to resume their normal functioning. Usually they still require daily dressing changes and nurses make certain that family members are taught how to assist the patient in dressing changes before being discharged. Also during this phase, patients are fitted with pressure garments that fit tightly over the healed skin to reduce scarring and disfiguration. Patients must return to the hospital periodically in the first year after discharge for occupational and physical therapy exercise and to check the progress of wound healing. After a years time, surgeons will determine other surgical needs of patients such as release of contractures (where skin has tightened to immobilize joints) or cosmetic procedures. Also at this time, the surgeons will make decisions about when normal activities and roles, particularly those related to work, can be resumed.

Having examined, however briefly, some of the problems that a burn injury presents to medical and nursing staffs, we can now proceed to look with more detail at the burn unit as a social setting.

The Burn Units

Both the adult and children's burn units were first and foremost areas of isolation and restricted space. Each of the units were located in areas of their respective hospitals that were physically removed from other wards where most patients and their families were likely to be found. Each of the two burn units were in the more quiet and remote regions of the hospital. Indeed, unless one were very familiar with these hospitals one would need directions to locate the burn units. While there were a few signs, the impression given was that the burn units were there for an extremely select group of patients, and their physical isolation discouraged random visiting and accidental intruders.

The doors leading into the burn units held impressively large signs that posted the visiting hours and the essential facts of visitation rights. Because burn patients were very vulnerable to infection, visitors were limited to immediate family and isolation procedures were adhered to. No one was allowed to enter either the children's or adult unit without donning a yellow cover gown to cover their street clothes. At the entrance to the units there was a large metal hamper filled with fresh cleaned yellow gowns and a smaller hamper for soiled gowns to be removed after leaving the unit. There were no exceptions to this rule for anyone and the nurses were diligent in getting people to conform.

Likewise, no one was allowed on the unit without a very specific reason. One had to be a family member, part of the medical or consulting staff or a visitor under special arrangements. One morning a young black woman simply wandered into a patient's room, lit up a cigarette and began a conversation. When the nurses realized she was a total stranger to the patient, security was called and she was quickly taken into custody for "possible criminal trespass."

While each burn unit was a relatively small area of space, the work performed on patients was defined as intensive and lifesaving. There were certain patient rooms reserved for the most severly burned and injured and these rooms contained sophisticated heart monitors and other machinery including video monitoring so that nurses could observe the patient's room from small television screens mounted in the nurses station and lounge.

Surgeons, nurses and therapists all wore surgical scrub suits which further defined the area as a critical care setting. There was a code-cart near each nursing station with resuscitation equipment and drugs for patients suffering cardiac or respiratory arrests. For patients and families, the code cart served as a reminder that not all patients would live and that part of what the staff does is to care for the dying.

The adult unit was physically laid out along a wide straight corridor of about forty yards. At the opposite end of the entrance to the burn unit was the hydrotherapy room, where patients were taken for their daily tankings and wound care. It was often a place of great pain for patients and interesting located farthest away from patient rooms, the nurses station and the television lounge. It was sealed off by two sets of heavy double doors.

Patients were assigned to one of nine individual rooms on either side of the hallway. Other rooms along the corridor included shower and bathrooms, the nurses station, the television lounge and several supply rooms. There was a small exercise area adjacent to the nurses station somewhat out of sight of the main hallway.

On some burn units in the United States burn patients are left "open" in that their wounds are covered only with topical antimicrobial dressings. This means that patients must stay isolated in their rooms and all staff and visitors entering their room must wear gowns, masks, hair nets and gloves. Unlike these burn units, the units I'm describing here use a "closed" technique in which white gauze dressings were wrapped over the topical creams and ointments. This allowed patients the freedom to leave their rooms without risk of infection and visitors need only to wear the protective cover gowns. Thus while there was a rather eerie silence on the burn units, nonetheless, one could see at least some of the patients in the adult unit out of bed, moving down the halls, or sitting in the lounge having a cigarette. Several patients were wrapped literally from head to toe and with their arms in splints that extended away from their torso, they made a ghost-like appearance.

Each patient was free to decorate her/his own room with greeting cards, letters from home and family pictures. However, the remainder of the adult burn unit was rather barren save for a number of inspirational posters taped along the hall. More will be said about their function in Chapter Four.

The children's unit contained seven beds in four rooms, that directly faced the nurses station. Three of the rooms had single beds for greater isolation, and one of those three was reserved for the most critical burn on the unit.

The atmosphere that prevailed on the children's unit was less restrictive and seemed less like a hospital. While the children were acutely burned, the unit was decorated to accentuate the physical surroundings as "kid space." There were large colorful mobiles and plastic airplanes suspended from the ceiling. Along one wall hung a series of toy shelves loaded with games, toys, puzzles and books. Except for at night and during nap time, those children who were well enough played among the toys that they often scattered along the floor in front of the nurses station. Parents and immediate family of burn children were allowed to visit on a twenty-four hour basis and they would sit in comfortable lounge chairs near the rooms playing with the children or reading them stories. Large colorful wagons sat in one corner and were used to transport children to therapy sessions or for play.

The Daily Routine

Every social setting has its own tempo and rhythm in which activities take place and events unfold. This is especially characteristic of hospital wards where daily routines of patient care are located in periods of time and space. So was the daily life of the burn units punctuated by the rhythm of activities and bounded by the space in which these activities were carried out.

The adult burn unit served at any time four to nine patients, the majority of whom were males and their ages ranged from seventeen to eighty years old. The modal patient was a male in his mid-twenties. For young, burned males, the restricted and isolated atmosphere of the burn unit made their experience all the more trying and difficult.

The daily round of caring for the burned began very early, the day shift nurses took over at 6:30 a.m. and nursing report was given at that time. Surgery residents and medical students normally drifted in around a half-hour later and proceeded to each patient's room to see how the night was spent. Though many patients had difficulty sleeping at night and some had only been asleep for a few hours, residents often woke them to see how they were feeling. If a patient was scheduled for surgery the resident would ask if there were any questions or related problems. Patients would awake blurry eyed, sometimes startled and confused and normally did not have any questions to ask. Some patients would mumble something to the effect that they weren't sleeping very well or that their pain medication wasn't working much. Since the residents had many other patients to see and were anxious on surgery days to get to the operating room, they didn't linger for long in the patient's room and if a patient had specific problems or complaints the resident would usually respond, "Well, we're going to look into that for you," and leave the room.

Each nurse was assigned daily to a patient sometimes more than one if the patient was not in critical condition. They would appear in the patient's room around 7:30 a.m. to check vital signs, administer medications and try to get the patient motivated to eat his/her breakfast. Though not all patients were hungry at this hour of the morning, many were required to take up to and exceeding 4,000 calories per day to promote wound healing, so that breakfast could not be skipped, though some patients would beg to do so.

For patients in the acute phase of wound healing the central event of the morning was their trip to the hydrotherapy tank for wound care and dressing changes. Nurses and physical therapists found this work activity consumed the greatest part of their morning and much of their physical and mental energy as well.

Since patients experience a good deal of pain during dressing changes, their nurses would administer pain medication about 20 minutes before their turn in the tank. Because of the limits of space and requirements of isolation to prevent infection, only one patient at a time could go to the tank room, thus each patient spent part of the morning waiting for his/her turn hoping that perhaps today the pain wouldn't be as bad as yesterday.

Patients were encouraged to walk to the tank room when they were able, but many were wheeled on a cart if still in the early critical phase. The tank room was large, but by ten o'clock in the morning its atmosphere was stuffy, hot and humid. On one side of the room sat the massive Hubbard tank which held many gallons of water, at the other side there was positioned a cart used for dressing changes and wound debridement. Any staff member in the tank room was required to wear gowns, gloves and masks as the patient's wounds would be fully exposed during these procedures.

In the morning hours the tank room was quite noisy with water splashing in the Hubbard, water pipes clanking and the radio playing a continuous stream of rock music. In the midst of this, nurses and the physical therapist would help each patient remove the gauze dressings, and then immerse the patient into the large tank of warm water. Once the patient became accustomed to the water temperature, the physical therapist would take up to ten minutes exercising the patient's arms and legs to prevent stiffness by loosening the muscles and skin over the joints. After the exercises, the burn wounds would be cleaned using small scrub pads. Patients were encouraged to do some of their own scrubbing on the chest and stomach areas that they could reach. During the cleansing, nurses would then take tweezers to pick at the dead burned skin on the wound, removing as must as they could each morning. As we will see in Chapter Four, all these activities just described could be extremely painful ordeals for patients.

After twenty minutes in the tank, patients were taken out and transferred to the dressing change cart for more wound debridement. This was followed by the dressing change itself which consisted of applying a fresh layer of antimicrobial medication to the wounds and fresh layers of gauze as a protective cover. During the time that the patient's wounds were exposed to the air, patients experienced a great deal of discomfort. They were quite relieved at the close of the dressing change when their wounds were once again sealed from the air. Dressing changes were often lengthy procedures, if a patient had a burn of over 50 percent surface area the entire dressing change could take up to two hours.

Patients often liked to return to their bed after dressing changes, hoping for a nap or rest before visiting hours at 11:00 a.m. However, Sandi, the occupational therapist found this period a good opportunity to exercise patients as their limbs and muscles were loose after hydrotherapy. On many mornings she would round up (almost literally) several ambulatory patients and steer them to the exercise area for a half hour of vigorous range of motion exercises.

Visiting on the adult unit was permitted from 11:00 a.m. to 2:00 p.m. and from 6:00 to 8:00 p.m. in the evening. Visitors were restricted to members of the immediate family and only two persons at a time could be in the patient's room. Visiting hours climaxed the morning's activities, it was the first glimpse each day of "outsiders," and brought the thickest density of people on the unit. This period also demarcated the end of the morning tanking and dressing changes which for some patients was their most painful part of the day. The unit was much quieter now, and patients looked forward to being left alone for awhile. After lunch and family visits they welcomed some nap time while the nurses busied themselves with their medication charts. Later, in the afternoon, however, the physical therapist would begin another round of exercises for each patient.

On the children's unit the rhythm was similar; early morning saw the residents making rounds and before noon most of the children were tubbed and had their dressings changed. Tanking, or "tubbing" as it was called on the children's unit, was done in one of two small rooms with large bathtubs in place of the Hubbard tank. Usually the tubs were loaded with rubber ducks and plastic toys to divert the child's attention. Families had unlimited visiting privileges and often parents slept in the rooms with their children on small hide-a-bed chairs. Some parents assisted with their child's wound care and dressing changes, primarily trying to soothe the child through the procedure. Other parents left the unit in the morning to get breakfast or to do laundry and would return at lunch time.

As on the adult unit, the noon hour signaled the end of the greatest flurry of activity and pain for children. Most of the screaming and shrieking were now over and the children, freshly scrubbed and bandaged, would noisily start pulling games and toys from the shelves and begin to play. With the arrival of lunch, however, anxieties began anew as many of the children didn't have much of an appetite and mealtime connoted for them another set of difficult expectations. Children would pick at their food while their parents and the nurses would coax, plead, threaten, bargain and use every trick in their arsenal to get them to eat. This contest would last up to an hour and usually ended with the parents getting upset and frustrated, as the children stubbornly won out, eating only half a hot dog and none of the vegetables or potatoes.

Children managed to get much of their exercise during their play periods, but at least once a day the physical or occupational therapist would show up to take those children who were ambulatory to the therapy department for exercise. On the children's unit much of the afternoon was considered nap time and lights were turned out, toys put away and the children were left alone to sleep. Most of the parents took this opportunity to leave the unit for a few hours to eat or take care of personal errands.

Grand Rounds

Burn patients, as we have seen, were treated in a variety of ways by members of the burn care team: surgeons, nurses, therapists and social workers. Sometimes team members worked alone, as a therapist might do in exercising a patient; other times they worked in tandem, when a nurse and therapist worked together debriding a patient's wound in the Hubbard tank; but in the rhythm of burn unit work there were two weekly occasions when all members of the team met and worked together in a visible and social sense. These occasions were referred to as Grand Rounds and Team Conference.

Grand Rounds were held every Monday morning at 8:00 a.m. in the adult unit and all members of the team were expected to be present. Rounds were conducted by the unit's medical director, a plastic surgeon, who supervised the work of the surgical residents.

One of the avowed purposes of Grand Rounds was to give the medical director and the residents together a chance to see all the patients "open." By "open" I mean, each patient had her/his dressings off so that the burn wounds could be directly inspected by the whole team, but especially by the surgeons since they were not able to see the wounds every day. For the nurses, Monday mornings were the height of their weekly activity since they were required to remove the dressings of every patient on the unit by 8:30 a.m. This was no small task and nurses usually had to help each other out as those patients with large burns required up to an hour just to get the dressings unwrapped!

According to the medical director, Grand Rounds afforded the team the opportunity to inspect each patient's wounds and physical condition, to mark signs of improvement and deterioration, to make judgments about the need for surgery and to decide which patients, if any, were ready to go home. In other words, Rounds would yield information whereby the staffs could make plans for each patient's course of treatment for the coming week. Sociologically, these were the stated or avowed functions of Grand Rounds. There were other functions or purposes of Grand Rounds which were not so explicitly recognized by staff and they included the following: patients often got information about their future, either directly or indirectly; and lower level staff such as nurses, therapists and social workers often gave information to surgeons and the medical director so that judgments could be made. Thus, Rounds were not simply inspection tours of burn wounds, they provided a structure for information exchange and a process whereby team members kept each other informed.

Grand Rounds began each Monday morning with the appearance of the medical director and without much of a greeting to the assembled staff, he would briskly move down the corridor to the first patient's room while the rest of the team hurriedly fell into place behind him, quickly tying on disposable masks over their hair nets. One got the feeling for medical hierarchy by participating in Grand Rounds, for each member of the team entered the patient's room according to her/his hospital status: the medical director entered first, followed by senior and junior surgical residents and medical students; the physicans were followed by the head nurse leading the nursing delegation, with the physical and occupational therapist pushing in closely behind. The burn unit social worker was the last of the team to enter the patient's room, and on her heels came the sociologist and any students thin enough to squeeze into a now crowded room. All of this rank ordering took only a few seconds as everyone knew their place. Since all those now assembled wore masks and hair coverings and considering that patients rarely saw the entire team together, this was a formidable picture for the patient. During Rounds there were no introductions to patients or indications of titles or purposes of the delegation. Patients who were on the unit for several weeks knew what to expect, new patients appeared bewildered and vulnerable.

There was not a great deal of verbal exchange among team members in front of the patient; that was reserved for the hallway after everyone had left the room. In lieu of introductions, the medical director proceeded to the head of a patient's bed and would say, "How are you doing this morning?" Then the inspection would begin. Rounds were "sight" work in that all staff considered their most important concern to be how the patient and her/his wounds looked. Thus everyone would gaze intently at the burn wounds, moving around the bed to get a better view all the while asking the patient to move in certain ways to expose the wounds more fully. The medical director would direct patients to "make a fist" or raise their arms above their head, as a way of testing range of motion. Some patients were lucky enough to draw praise if their skin grafts were taking or if their skin was healing in quickly or if it was obvious to the surgeons that they had been exercising and had good range of motion in their limbs.

Grand Rounds were especially important to the physical and occupational therapists, as a patient's ability to show improvement in range of motion was a reflection on their skills in working with patients. They wanted their patients to do well in front of the medical director, but often patients failed to live up to expectations because hands and joints became dry and stiff shortly after the dressings were removed and patients were stiffest in the early morning hours. The therapists tried encouraging the patients to do their best. The following took place one morning on Rounds:

Medical Director: "John, can you make a fist with that left hand?"
John (a 19 year old male): After some feeble and unsuccessful attempts, "I guess I just can't."
Sandi (occupational therapist): "Oh yes you can John, now come on!"
Medical Director: After glancing at Sandi, "Well John, looks to me like you got lazy over the weekend."

The medical director occasionally handed out praise to the surgery residents on their successes. "That graft really looks good." "Oh, this is coming along very nice." Nurses were often asked what topical creams or ointments they were using on certain wounds and there would be occasional suggestions from the director to try different types of dressings.

Patients often wanted information about their progress or future. However, Rounds took place at a fairly brisk pace and the anonymity of these encounters was heightened by the masks, thus, most patients didn't ask questions nor were they encouraged to. Many patients appeared intimidated by the crowd around their bed and as their wounds were very painful without the gauze dressings, patients were much too uncomfortable to be talkative or inquisitive. Although there were times during Rounds when patients were told they would need more surgery or for the more fortunate ones, that their wounds had healed to the point that they could go home.

After the patient's wounds were thoroughly inspected, the entire team would retire from the room to the hall where the medical director lead a discussion of the patient's condition. During these discussions, decisions were made about the possible need for additional surgery or medication changes. Also there were attempts to ascertain how close some patients were to going home or in the opposite extreme, how near some patients were to death. On some occasions, the medical director did some more formal type of teaching, leading the residents and anyone else who cared to listen through an analysis of a particular disease entity and its medical management. These hallway meetings lasted only a few minutes, but did provide nurses and therapists a chance to ask the medical director about decisions they had to make and also to give him information about the more subtle changes in the condition and behaviors of the patient just seen. With a few minutes the next patient was descended upon.

Grand Rounds on the children's unit were not nearly so formal and structured and were conducted even more briefly. There was no entourage effect. Rounds were made by the medical director, surgical residents, medical students and perhaps a nurse or two. Rounds were held at 8:30 a.m. on Mondays and the physicians moved quickly from room to room. As usual, they wore masks and hair nets and made no introductions of themselves to new patients or their families. In the most restricted sense, these Rounds were for wound inspection only. Parents generally were not talked to, nor were explanations given to them about the purpose of Rounds, nor about the decisions at which the surgeons might ultimately arrive. The physicians looked only at the burn wounds and even limited their exchanges with each other solely to that topic. It was assumed that the children had little comprehension of what was being discussed, several times children learned of their impending surgery as the medical director issued orders to that effect to the residents. Little was said directly to the children and they were not given the opportunity ask questions or express their fears about surgery — at least during Grand Rounds.

After all the children had been seen, the medical director normally sought out the charge nurse to ask her if there were any problems he needed to know about and they would discuss briefly the surgical decisions he had made and she, in turn, would indicate which of the children the nursing staff felt were ready to go home. This discussion essentially signaled the completion of Rounds on the children's unit.

Team Conference

Team conferences are common among burn centers in the United States, though their form and name will vary. They are usually weekly or monthly meetings where all members of the burn care team meet to discuss as a group the recovery of each patient currently on the unit. In this study, team meetings were thought to be necessary in that each member of the team could share with others how their particular responsibilities toward the patient were being carried out and what problems, if any, they were encountering. The weekly team conferences were different from Grand Rounds in that patients were not directly visible to the staff and the discussions of patient progress was not limited solely to the nature of the patient's physical recovery. In team conference, patients were evaluated much more broadly, not simply in terms of their physical well-being, but, also, their emotional status, willingness to comply with the demands of the patient role, relationships with family and a number of other behavioral concerns. Team conference, then, was a broad but not necessarily lengthy discussion of the current state of each patient on the unit. Also, since team conferences were held in a conference room away from the unit, it afforded members of the burn unit an opportunity to relax, loosen up and engage, at least for

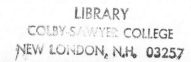

a few minutes, in less serious behavior and demeanor. As we shall see, while team conference was taken seriously and considered an important part in the work of the burn unit staff, there was usually some sociability and even humorous exchange before, during and after the conference. Part of the sociability and humor was due to the awkwardness staff felt in coming together away from the unit and out of sight from the patients. There was no direct "hands on" work to do here and staff found themselves uncomfortably looking at each other in a semi-circle of chairs. The one thing that staff had in common, the patient, was not physically present, and the patient was to be "discussed," not examined or cared for. This was not an easy task for a staff that preferred and even thrived on a more activist orientation toward patient care. Thus, the attempts at lighthearted sociability and good natured joking and kidding was a way of overcoming that awkwardness of meeting in a formal conference.

Team meetings were attended by the medical director, the head nurse, the social worker, the occupational and physical therapists, mental health consults, the chaplain and representatives from the microbiology lab. The medical director viewed the team conferences as a vehicle for keeping him abreast of the progress of each patient. Thus while team conferences ideally were a democratic sharing of concerns and information about patients, in actuality, much of the discussion was directed toward the medical director for his approval. However, the medical director did not chair the meetings, this was the responsibility of the head nurse, who introduced each patient's history for discussion. Interestingly, even when some patients had been on the unit for over two months, their cases were introduced very formally, as if the team were hearing about the person for the first time. The following is taken from field notes on a fairly typical team conference on the adult burn unit:

> Team conference began a few minutes late today as the Dr. Williams, the unit medical director, came directly from surgery. The usual group was present: Audry, the head nurse; Chaplain La Forge; Betty, the social worker, Sandi and Peg, the occupational and physical therapists, and two women from the microbiology lab. Dr. Williams, the medical director, walked in about 1:15 still dressed in his surgical scrubs with a white lab coat.
>
> Dr. Williams: "Well, Father La Forge is here — now you can't

pick on me!" Everyone in the room laughed.

Sandi: "I've got a student with me today — Jean Harris and I'll be supervising her practicum in occupational therapy." Everyone smiled in her direction. Audry, the head nurse started abruptly on the first patient for discussion. She read from a card.

Audry: "Randy O'Conner, is a seventeen year old male, who was admitted on the fifteenth of June. He had a brain injury and sustained twenty-five percent full thickness burns to his legs and right side."

Dr. Williams: "He still has it."

Audry: "Isn't that what I just said?"

Dr. Williams: "I thought you said he *had* a brain injury on June fifteenth. He still *has* the brain injury." This was followed by laughter around the room.

Audry: "I see — yes, indeed, Ah . . . Randy still has a brain injury and he also has positive blood cultures."

Dr. Williams, looking at the microbiologist: "Where is it coming from?"

Microbiologist: "We didn't divide it up." (This meant that microbiology didn't differentiate whether the infection was from his burn wound or his head injury.)

Dr. Williams: "Well . . . I guess we won't operate on him tomorrow."

Audry: "Do you have any kind of feeling, Dr. Williams, on how he's going to do?"

Dr. Williams: "I have no way of giving a prognosis on him, but my gut reaction is that it's awful. He's got a 25 percent full thickness burn injury, a pulmonary injury . . . and a cerebral injury."

Team conference not only set benchmarks on patient's recovery and progress, but also included discussions of who was ready to go home and whether the family was prepared to care for the patient in the home. Family dynamics were thought to be special province of the social worker, who normally had little to say in team conferences, unless the medical director wanted her assessment of a particular family's ability to cope or come to terms. She was then expected to have information readily available concerning the resources of the family and their willingness and capacity to provide adequate and responsible home care if the patient was discharged.

Team conference was also an occasion for staff members to get emotional release from the tensions and anxieties associated with working on acutely ill and dying patients. Many of the patients discussed in team conference were horribly injured, suffering tremendous physical pain and facing death. It was not easy for burn staff to work on these patients and it was even more difficult to discuss their injuries and conditions in detached and neutral terms. Each level of staff felt these stresses and anxieties in their own ways, but one of the coping devices employed in common was the use of humor as a way of coming to terms. Humor became the vehicle for dealing with staff anxieties about burn work and a way of facing the uncertainties in medical judgment and decision-making. Humor allowed the team to approach and recognize their own fears and uncertainties in a way the rational, serious, technical discourse would not.

One area of uncertainty in medical treatment had to do with infection or sepsis which was the leading cause of death among burn patients. Despite the staff's rigid adherence to isolation procedures and sterile technique, not all infection causing bacteria could be controlled, and many patients succumbed to infection after being on the unit for several weeks. Another area of uncertainty surrounded those patients with multiple disease problems in addition to their burn injury, which complicated tremendously the treatment of the burn. Almost in despair such cases were approached through humor as a way of coping. Here are two short examples from team conferences:

> Devon (the bacteriologist) to Dr. Williams: "By the way . . . what about that bug that was resistant to everything we tried? How did you get rid of it?"
> Dr Williams: "We didn't. The patient died and it died with him."
> Audry: "At least we hope it did!"
> Dr. Williams, smiling: "Yes . . . we certainly hope so."

> Audry: "Let's begin with Fred Jones. He is a seventy-six year old male with 50 percent partial thickness burns. He is on a respirator . . . He has cancer of the stomach and a history of heart trouble and emphysema. He had a heart attack two months prior to his burn. Oh! . . . and he also has a glass eye. Dr. Williams — what should we do with that?"
> Dr. Williams, looking at Audry: "Polish it!"

The weekly team conferences on the children's unit included the same team roles; physicians, nurses, therapists, etc., but of course, not the same people. In contrast with the adult unit, team conferences were often held in the absence of the medical director though on occasion one of the surgical residents would attend. Also, by way of contrast, since the families of the children were such a presence on the ward and considered to be instrumental in the emotional support necessary for children to recover from burn injuries, much of the discussion here in team conference centered around the adequacy of parents and their strength or lack of parenting skills and the consequent behavior problems of their children. There were usually a number of mental health and child psychology consultants attending team conference and in addition to the talk about wound management, nutrition and range of motion problems there was much ado about the emotional coping skills of parents and children. Much of the discussion about parents and children was evaluative in substance and heavily psychological in explanation and interpretation.

Nurses in team conference were most concerned with what they considered the inappropriate behavior of children: not eating, temper tantrums, excessive demands and vocal excesses in pain expression. With respect to the latter, for example, nurses expected children to scream during debridement of the wounds, but *not* when the child was merely sitting in the tub and not being touched. Nurses were also concerned with the parenting skills of the mothers and fathers and expected their support in getting the children to comply with the program. So strong was the need to make parents a part of the recovery program, that when parents were talked about they were referred to as "Mom" and "Dad," not as "the Mom" or "her Mom."

In team conference many of the nursing staff frustrations with parent's lack of support or inability to cope responsibly became central to the discussion. Parents were discussed as much as the children! The medical director and surgery residents, when in attendance, remained aloof from these topics, and they tended to limit their remarks to strictly medical and surgical problems or prognosis. Thus team conference on the children's unit tended to divide up between the science — oriented male surgeons whose primary concern was the patient's medical/surgical needs; and the nurture-oriented female nurses and psychology consultants (also women) whose concerns primarily were with the emotional health or inadequacies of the children and their parents.

Partly as a result of this divergence in interest and concern, physicians were often absent from team meetings and were the least vocal of the participants. I've included a brief excerpt from one team meeting to give the reader an idea of the dynamics. Lydia, the child being referred to, was a two and a half year old female, who had full thickness scald burns to her legs and trunk.

> Georgia (nurse): "Well . . . we're still having problems with Lydia who cries and screams all the time. She started screaming yesterday and all I did was take her temperature for God's sake!"
>
> Doris (mental health clinician): "It sound like her way of getting attention. It probably got her what she wanted before and she's doing it now. She knows you'll give in . . . She's probably acted the same way with Mom."
>
> Edna (child guidance consultant): "I wonder if Mom and Dad are consistent with her. I know Dad isn't around much and Lydia seems to have Mom wrapped around her finger. Mom will get angry with her for doing something and then later when Lydia does it again — Mom won't say a word! I just wonder if Mom was ever in control of that child!"
>
> Doris: "You might try some behavior mod with her. Maybe that would work."

Such discussions often continued for sometime with the surgeons standing silently in the background. Occasionally a question would be directed their way and one of the residents would nod in agreement or briefly interject a comment or two. Little was ever completely resolved in children's team conference; consultants suggested techniques for nurses to try, or promised to pay closer attention to the child for further evaluation. Team conferences had mostly a cathartic effect for burn nurses who felt a need to vent their frustrations in working so closely and intimately with burned children and their parents. If nothing was ever settled, for most nurses it seemed enough that these issues were vigorously and thoroughly discussed in "team."

Having looked at some of the daily routines and weekly events in the burn care setting it is now necessary to examine more closely the roles that comprise the burn team. Since the nurses were most heavily involved in the day to day care of burn patients and spent the most time in their treatment, I'll begin with them.

Nursing the Burned Patient

When burned patients recovered from their injuries and were convalescing at home, some of their most vivid recollections of their hospital experiences were about the nurses who took care of them. When surgical residents began a three month rotation on the burn unit, they anticipated that their success in coping with the demands of that rotation would be related to their ability to work smoothly and efficiently with the burn unit nurses. Of the entire burn care team, it was often the nurses who had worked on the unit the longest and had chosen to work in a burn unit.

Nursing care of the burn patient was a twenty-four hour a day responsibility; nurses spent the most time in the physical presence of burn patients and as a result came to know the most about them. Because of this, burn nurses tended to think possessively about the burn unit, often referring to it as "our unit."

In their twenty-four hour a day care for burn patients, nurses carried out a number of activities that formed the core of that role. Nurses devised care plans for patients, followed surgeon's orders on medications and lab tests and monitored critical patients attached to suction, ventilators, hear monitors, etc. Burn unit nursing was considered above all, critical or intensive care nursing. In addition, nurses were responsible for keeping meticulous charts detailing the conditions of their patients and the various treatments and procedures administered to them.

Aside from these critical care functions, burn unit nurses thought themselves to be the wound care specialists. When new nurses were being taught "the ropes" as a burn care nurse, they were given many hours of instruction, both formal and informal about burn wounds: what they look like, how to look for signs of infection and healing, how to treat them, etc. Much of the daily routine of the nurses was taken up in caring for burn wounds and when nurses discussed the progress of the patients for whom they were responsible the stuff of the conversation was about how the wounds looked. For a nurse to be "up" on a patient, that is to be familiar with the patient's condition, was essentially to be familiar with the wound. When a nurse said, "I haven't seen Tom in a few days," she meant she hadn't seen his burn wound.

Burn nurses saw wounds daily as they took their assigned patients to the tank, cleansed and debrided the burn wounds and put on clean dressings. In this sense, much of the nurse's work was "visual," it was treating a wound, but equally important it was seeing the wound, evaluating it's condition, and passing this information on to the surgeons so that decisions could be made with regard to further treatment. Nurses evaluated their work in terms of their ability to get wounds to "heal in" and in this domain they assumed a good deal of latitude in daily wound care. While the surgery residents wrote the medication orders for wound care nurses often suggested to them which procedures might work best and within those general orders, nurses innovated trying different combinations of dressings and ointments, and debriding techniques. Burn nurses argued that experience was the best judge in matters of wound care and usually persuaded the residents to go along with their more seasoned and experienced judgments.

Among other nursing responsibilities was to reinforce the treatment programs of the physical and occupational therapists. Thus, nurses also became concerned with patient's range of motion progress, their ability to do for themselves in activities of daily living, and patient compliance in areas of physical exercise, splint wearing and use of pressure garments. As we shall examine more closely in subsequent chapters, part of the nurses responsibility was to be a psychological motivator of their patients in getting them to accept the demands inherent in their recovery. This meant that a burn unit nurse had to be demanding and willing to push patients to their limits of physical pain and endurance. In this aspect, nurses had to confront most directly how this part of their role was so at odds with their views of themselves as nurturers and comforters. Nurses were continually faced with the fact that their work caused patients to be in pain and discomfort, and they were limited in their ability to ease the patient's burden. Unlike traditional nursing with its emphasis on nurturing and comforting patients, burn nurses had to accept a definition of the nursing role as a pain inflicter and enforcer of a set of rigorous demands on patients to endure and tolerate their pain.

One of the Head Nurses in an interview described burn nursing in this way:

> J.M.: "Can a burn nurse do her/his job if she/he is not a 'pusher'?"
>
> H.N.: "No — when I interview people (prospective nurses) that is one of the things I stress — how do you feel as a pain inflicter? If you can't divorce yourself from the idea that the patient is angry with you now . . . but in a month or two down the road when the patient goes home — that is when the reward is going to come. If you need that instant gratification and your role is that of a nurturer — well that's not what a burn nurse does. If you want your patients to like you, the burn unit is not the place to be. It's only much later they (patients) cry on your shoulder and tell you how wonderful you are."

Because of their responsibilities as pain inflicters and given the fact that many of their patients die or recover in slow and agonizing ways nurses looked for ways to bolster their morales and enhance their solidarity as nurses on the unit. In trying to gain a measure of distance from the more disagreeable aspects of their role, nurses sought to maintain a sense of togetherness and bondedness that supported them in times of stress and difficulty. They attempted to unify and present an image of a solid front as a way of coming to terms. For example, sociability among nurses was considered very important as a mechanism of mutual support and team centeredness. Social relations among nurses were quickly upgraded; newly hired nurses were eagerly embraced into the group by encouraging a first name basis, learning each other's biographies, sharing food at lunch and dinners, and remembering birthdays. In fact, on both the children's and adult unit it was though to be a breach of etiquete to neglect someone's birthday. Birthdays for each month were marked on a large calender on the adult unit and painted on a window in the children's unit. Birthdays were vigorously celebrated with cakes, special foods, humorous cards and gifts.

On the children's unit there was a large poster board on the wall in the nursing lounge and each month was a theme depicting the nurses (and surgery residents) in some sort of construction paper cut-out. During the month of May, the 500 Mile Race was the theme and under a slogan, "You're never in the Pits with the BUNS" (burn unit nurses), there was portrayed a race track with small paper cars, each one labeled with a nurse's name. In June, the theme was picnic and each nurse was a construction paper hamburger and the residents' were hot dogs.

In their work roles, burn nurses were expected to be toughminded, no-nonsense types; strict enforcers of the often painful and agonizing requirements of a burn patient's recovery. Yet, in their informal relations with fellow nurses, they worked hard to maintain some distance from that role by promoting an aura of sociability, tenderness, and non-serious demeanors of birthday parties, lunch time gossip and arts and crafts.

Newly hired nurses were socialized into the role of a burn nurse during a long process of orientation. Most new nurses were recent nursing school graduates who wanted to work in a critical care setting because of the challenges they perceive. Many elected to work with burn patients and that set them apart from most nurses who distain that career and served to immediately ingratiate them with the experienced burn unit staff because it validated for them the importance of their work.

Orientation of new nurses was long and arduous. Since critical care nursing involved the learning of many complicated techniques and procedures, new nurses were given several weeks of freedom in which they mostly observed the work of experienced nurses. In the area of wound care, only after some weeks were new nurses given small and uncomplicated dressing changes to do on their own.

Some of their orientation was more formal and consisted of slide picture demonstrations given by an experienced nurse, on the various nursing procedures involved in critical burn care. Interestingly, several of these slides contained some of the goriest pictures of burn wound; including pictures of patients whose bodies were virtually charred and slides of amputations resulting from electric burns. New nurses often cringed at these sights while the orientation nurse calmly and with great detachment continued her lecture on the physiology of the wound. The purpose of those slides appeared to be twofold: to instruct nurses about wound care and to desensitize them to the graphic ugliness of burn wounds.

One recently hired nurse on the children's unit had finished several weeks of orientation and was asked to assist one of the staff nurses in debriding the wound of a young boy who had massive scald wounds and blisters covering his buttocks. After a few minutes in the patient's room she hurried out complaining of dizziness and nausea, and had to sit down for awhile in the nurses lounge. She later explained to me, "I thought I was prepared to look at things like that, but when I actually saw his butt, it almost made me sick! I felt better after I rested for awhile."

New nurses also had to come to terms with their roles as a pain inflicter. Many inexperienced nurses were disturbed about hurting patients during wound debridement and dressing changes, and they tried initially to be as gentle and tender as they could. They would often apologize to patients for having caused them pain. For these reasons, many patients looked forward to having one of the newly hired nurses assigned to them. They knew that these nurses would be more solicitous, careful, and proceed much more slowly in doing dressing changes. Thus, student and new nurses were often the most popular and well liked among the patients. The experienced nurses recognized this fact and it seemed not to bother them, as if they remembered their earliest days on the unit and their own squeamishness and reluctance to cause discomfort. These nurses expected that their less experienced colleagues would soon toughen up to the job.

As not all burn patients would live through their ordeal, nurses also had to deal with the reality of losing patients. This problem was especially acute in the burn units, where the dying patient was often young. Moreover, since most burn patients died of infection induced by the burn injury, they did not always die in the first few days of their admission. In fact, several patients in this study died slow, lingering deaths weeks after they were successfully resuscitated in the critical or emergent phase. Such patients regained consciousness, became ambulatory and survived several surgeries only to die of infection a month or so after being admitted.

This proved difficult for nurses because during that period the patients became part of the social web of the unit: they had an identity, a biography and a family with whom nurses would have become involved. In this sense, the social death of the patient was more trying for the nurses and staff than the biological death. I'm reserving a more detailed account of work among the dying for a later chapter.

Having looked at the role of the burn nurse it is now time to turn our attention to her/his most immediate ally but occasional adversary in burn care; the burn surgeon.

The Burn Surgeon

The ultimate medical responsibility for burn patients was in the hands of the burn surgeon. As in all hospital medicine, the physican was the final authority and was legally responsible for the medical decisions, thus, the burn unit was no exception. On both the children's and adult units, the surgeon wrote the orders for procedures and medical interventions for patients and the rest of the team carried them out.

Burn surgeons worked within a rather rigid hierarchy of physician status arrangements. The adult burn unit and the children's unit were each under the medical supervision of a plastic surgeon, each of whom were hospital staff physicians in the Department of Plastic Surgery. Furthermore, each of these surgeons held professorships in the University School of Medicine. These men supervised the work of six senior residents in plastic surgery. These senior residents were in their final two years of a prolonged residence in surgery which included five years in general surgery. Each plastic surgery resident served a three month rotation through the two burn units as part of that plastic surgery residency. During that 3 month rotation, the senior resident was responsible for making most of the medical and surgical judgments on patients in the burn units. The senior resident was assisted by a general surgery resident doing an elective two month rotation in plastic surgery, and varying numbers of junior and senior medical students doing 1 month electives in surgery.

Both burn units, like many others in the United States, served two functions: education and patient care. The two burn units provided surgery residents opportunities to learn techniques for plastic and reconstructive surgery within a mandate to care for critically burned patients. As we shall see later, these two functions were at times at odds with one another and had significant implications for what was referred to as the team approach to burn treatment. In supervising the work of the senior residents, one of the medical directors explained the arrangement in the way, "Some burn units in the United States have full time surgeons and that is their sole responsibility. But, here you're dealing with an academic institution. Part of my job is to direct the energy of residents to learn how to care for burned patients. But, the decision is ultimately mine. The better the resident the more latitude he'll have in directing care. Whatever he wants to delegate to the general surgery resident is fine. But if anything goes wrong, its the senior resident that I'm going after."

In the daily activities of the burn units, the surgery residents made the medical judgments about patient care, however, physically they were not present in the burn unit for more than an hour or two each day. Residents made patient rounds daily around 7:00 a.m., but this normally took less than twenty minutes. Tuesdays, Thursdays and Fridays were "surgery days" and residents spent most of their time in the operating room doing surgery on burn patients and other patients on the hospital's plastic surgery service. Wednesday was clinic day in which the residents examined, on an out-patient basis, all the patients released from the burn unit and who were now recuperating at home. Residents normally would be on hand to help with a new burn admission, and when they wanted to closely examine a patient's burn wounds when the patient was "open" they often made brief morning appearances in the therapy tank room. Because of the relatively limited amount of time residents spent with burn patients, they depended a great deal on the information nurses and therapists provided for them about patients' medical conditions and physical and psychological progress. Thus, partly by the constraints of their busy surgery schedules and their responsibilities to other hospital services, residents were pulled into the team matrix by their dependency on the kind of information about patients that only burn nurses and therapists could provide.

Burn surgeons were interested in the overall recovery of patients, they could often be heard remarking how important it was to send a man or woman home to family and community as soon and as healed as possible. In this respect, they shared the same goals as other members of the team. However, their more immediate, practical concerns were with the physical/medical problems of their patients. As might be expected, surgeons tended to view burn care from the standpoint of the patient's surgical needs, liabilities and potentials. In the view of one burn surgeon, "Our (surgeons) problems fall into two categories, I would say. First of all, we have-to have a patient who is *alive* to work with. During the acute phase we are trying to create a stable patient. For example, stabilizing a lung status or other trauma related problem the patient might have. After that is accomplished, and *if* it is accomplished, we are faced with the reconstructive aspect. Based on our assessment of the burn wound injury — how can we maximize a patient's aesthetic and functional result back to society? We're not even concerned with the psychology at this point. We want to get the wound closed as expeditiously as possible with the best quality of skin coverage as we can."

Thus, much of the work of the burn unit physician could be understood from the nature of burn injury trauma in general, and from practical surgical decisions and judgments in particular. The critically burned presented a significant medical if not surgical challenge to the physicians, and this challenge colored and to a certain degree dominated how surgeons viewed the recovery process.

Because the care of burn patients was entrusted to residents in plastic surgery, surgery took on special meanings. For residents, surgery was always an opportunity to get practice in making medical judgments and to gain clinical experience. However, from the viewpoint of plastic surgery residents, surgery on burn patients was not very rewarding, as cosmetically pleasing outcomes were rarely forthcoming. While residents did gain some opportunities for cosmetic reconstructive surgery on burn patients, in fact, the bulk of their work was limited to excising burn wounds, laying skin grafts and surgical release of contractures. Several residents expressed their frustration that these procedures did not take much surgical skill and were not the kind of surgeries that would prepare them for their later work in private practice. One senior resident expressed it this way, "This place (hospital) can be a zoo. There's not much chance for cosmetic surgery. There you are standing up to your ankles in blood and you're just trying to get him covered and off the table before he gets cold . . . just get him covered as quickly as you can."

Skin grafting itself as a surgical procedure did not reflect on the skills of the plastic surgeon, which also frustrated some of the residents. Another surgery resident told me, "Even when you think you have done a good job the day of the graft it might not look good a year later. However, if you have done a shitty graft — you know it will never look any better! No plastic surgeon brags about grafts on burn patients. Plastics want to make people look better than they did before. But in burns — you're just covering up!" The burn unit medical director realized this dilemma that seems to be unavoidable in surgery on burn patients. Here is a quote from our interview.

> Medical Director: "We know that senior residents don't like skin grafting. They like to hand it down. (To the general surgery resident.) If it goes well — it should go well. When it doesn't, it's someone else's fault. But you know, the residents never get to see the patients come back. The residents are on the unit for only a few months. They don't get to see the patients a year or so later being rehabilitated back into society in the functional aspect."

For surgery residents, a rotation on the burn unit was also fraught with the dilemmas that arose from their lack of experience in treating burn wounds. Since they were essentially plastic surgeons their exposure to burn wound trauma was usually limited. As a result, they often found themselves in the awkward situation of being the ultimate medical authority over patients whose conditions they had little direct and practical experience in treating! This made their situation especially vulnerable to burn unit nurses, many of whom had years of experience in treating and caring for burn wounds. Thus, in both burn units there was often considerable friction between the nurses who were clinically experienced, but with limited medical authority, taking orders from surgeons who were legally and medically responsible but were clinical novices in burn wound care. This is not to say that there were not other areas in the medical recovery of burn patients where the surgeons knowledge was superior, recognized and crucial. But in the area of the burn wound itself, nurses considered their knowledge superior and in many subtle and not-so-subtle ways encouraged the residents to recognize this. Such grudging recognition by residents was usually forthcoming. As one senior resident expressed it, "The nurses run the show — and any resident who thinks he is any more than a consultant is fooling himself. Sure we give the orders and do the surgery, but the nurses take

care of the patients — they know what to do! When I was an intern
on a burn unit several years ago, I didn't know shit about burns. But
when a patient came in, the nurses went to the emergency room,
evaluated him and handed me the protocol and told me what the orders should be! It was only after I had been there awhile and learned
that they begin to value my medical opinion."

Despite this mixture of medical authority and clinical inexpe-
rience, nurses could not "run the show" as this resident lamented.
The surgeons still gave the orders, made the surgical decisions, and
ultimately decided which patients would stay and which would go
home. The work of the nurse was much more constrained by the
medical authority of the surgeon than was usually admitted, and this
phenomenon placed severe strains on the team concept of burn care.
We will examine the dynamics of these strains between nurses and
residents when we look more closely at the recovery, and dying trajectories in subsequent chapters. For now, there remains other
members of the burn care team to be introduced.

Physical and Occupational Therapy

Physical and occupational therapists also become significantly involved in treating burn patients, although the scope of their work
varies among burn units in the United States. For example, on the
adult unit being examined here, the physical and occupational
therapists spent several hours a day on the unit working with patients and their daily presence formed a definite part of the web of
social relationships with the rest of the staff. Conversely, on the children's unit, the therapists appeared only when their services were
immediately needed and at those times that the nurse requested
their help. The scope of their activities on the children's unit also appeared to be limited.

On the adult unit, physical therapists engaged in a variety of activities in treating the burned. The several therapists assigned to the
unit were women and usually in their late twenties and early thirties,
which gave them a close age and gender compatibility with the nursing staff. Their duties included involvement in wound care, thus on
the adult unit most of their mornings were spent in the tank room assisting the nurses with wound debridement and dressing changes. In
addition, the physical therapist was responsible for exercising pa-

tients to minimize deformity, restore muscle functions, and to maintain range of motion in the patient's limbs. Much of the work of the therapist was conducted in the large hydrotherapy tank when the patient's muscles and joints were loosened in the warm water.

Burned skin tightens and contracts and when skin is burned over joints such as elbows, shoulders, and wrists, a patient can lose range of motion and can quickly become virtually immobilized through inability to stretch and bend their limbs. These conditions are referred to as contractures and the goal of the therapists was to prevent contractures by leading patients through daily programs of physical exercise. Patients often found these exercises very painful and uncomfortable because they were, in effect, attempting to stretch burned skin that was raw, sore and sensitive. It was the physical therpists lot that most if not all the work they did for patients was pain inducing.

As a result, therapists became concerned with the psychological motivation of their patients to "work through" their pain and endure the exercises the therapists considered necessary to insure physical mobility. One therapist told me that these concerns became paramount when she made her initial assessments of patients.

> Therapist: "Now I look at the total size of the patient . . . and what kind of personality they have. Are they athletic? Are they motivated to do exercises or do I have to motivate them? What kind of approach do I have to take? Am I going to have to get them to do something they haven't done in twenty years?
>
> J.M.: "How do you get patients to do what you want them to do?"
>
> Therapist: "Lots of bargaining! I set a goal they can reach — a lot less than they are capable of. People will comply with a goal they know about. Even if they vocalize a lot of pain — I don't stop. Though I wouldn't push just to get my way. I operate on this premise: If I was the one burned, I would want someone to push me even if I beg.
>
> Many patients have told me they don't remember how awful the agony was the first few weeks. Well, that's compensation for me — I just hope they don't remember it and I go ahead with what needs to be done."

In light of this, some physical therapists tended to lessen the burden they feel as pain inducers, by emphasizing the role they played in their empathetic response to patients. The following is taken from an interview with a therapist who had worked in several burn units in the United States:

> J.M.: "What is the most important thing you do for patients in your daily routines?"
>
> Therapist: "Listening to them! I think I spend more time with patients than anyone else. Sometimes a whole hour of uninterrupted time. More time than even the nurses. Granted that the dresssing changes take a long time but they usually involve several nurses and they are chaotic. You wouldn't tell several nurses what you would tell someone alone. Patients tell me things because the nurses are busy. The nurse has a lot of things to do every day. But a therapist has only one thing — exercise patients. And patients can talk during an exercise routine and I listen to their concerns!"

The work of the occupational therapist overlaps somewhat with that of physical therapy, in that occupational therapy is also concerned with restoring muscle function. In the adult unit, the occupational therapist did not get involved in the daily tubbings, but lead each patient through a round of exercises to restore and maintain range of motion. In conjunction with that, the occupational therapist was responsible for devising splints which attached to a patient's limb to minimize deformity and were positioned in such a way to enhance range of motion. These therapists told me that their motto, or professional credo was, "The Position of Comfort is the Position of Deformity." Thus, while splinting of limbs and joints was therapeutically necessary, patients found such positioning painful. In the emergent phase, these splints were worn continuously, but during the acute phase they were worn only at night and at rest periods. Patients lamented that if they had their way, they wouldn't be worn at all!

The occupational therapists in this study attended all team conferences and Grand Rounds, and provided nurses and surgeons with much information about patient's progress in terms of their ability to ambulate, feed themselves, and engage in other activities of daily living. In fact, when making judgments toward the end of a patient's recovery trajectory concerning their ability to return home or to work, the opinions of the physical and occupational therapists were considered to be of great value. Surgeons often postponed sending a patient home if the therapists felt that a patient needed more "work" in being able physically to do for themselves.

Nevertheless, while physical and occupational therapy were considered a part of the team and had daily responsibilities in caring for patients, they did not have the kind of authority in matters of medical judgment as did the surgeons and nurses. In this sense, their domain of authority was restricted to the motor activities of patients, which limited their mandate in being able to make more comprehensive judgments and decisions about the course of a patient's treatment. This seemed especially the case on the children's unit where the physical therapist did not assist in the daily tubbings and wound care and visited the unit only once a day to take the children off the unit for their exercise sessions. On both burn units, surgeons and nurses tended to define their responsibilities for patient care much more broadly and assumed a greater latitude in authority and decision-making. It can be argued then that the burn unit was the domain of the nursing and surgical services and other members of the team found their range of authority in patient care much more restricted.

Social Work

Burn unit social workers occupied an interesting position on the burn care team in that they were non-medical personnel and took no direct part in the medical care of patients. Their role was defined largely in terms of the work they did in helping patients and families come to terms with the many social, economic, and psychological problems that arose in their hospital and posthospital recovery.

Each burn unit employed its own social worker, both of whom were women, and while their general responsibilities toward patients were similar, there were specific differences in each of their approaches that were influenced by the differences inherent in working with child and adult patients.

On the children's unit, the social worker spent much of the time with parents and families of patients assisting them with the variety of problems they faced. This included helping them cope with the family strains associated with having a child undergoing a prolonged hospitalization. She also gave advice and counsel to parents about obtaining financial assistance in paying for the child's considerable hospital expenses and other costs incurred by parents in making living and housing arrangements near the hospital for a lengthy stay. In addition, the social worker assumed liaison relationships between the burn unit and external authorities in cases of child abuse and neglect which occurred with some frequency. In this capacity she kept the burn unit staff informed about the nature and current state of police and child welfare investigations into suspected cases. As she acquired a good deal of information about the background of parents and families of burn children, she took an active and vocal role in the weekly team conferences in which the staff gathered to discuss the progress of each child. During team conference she carefully informed the staff relative to how each parent and family was adjusting to having their child on the unit, especially in terms of their psychological adjustment, and she also provided information to the staff about the status of any child abuse investigation that might have been going on. In contrast to the social worker on the adult unit, she spent less time talking to the children, as many of them were in the pre-verbal age group.

The adult unit social worker spent relatively equal time talking and counseling with both patients and families. During the emergent phase, the first few days of a patient's hospitalization, she met frequently with the family helping them secure temporary housing, if required, and assuring and informing them about the critical care procedures being carried out on the patient. Many families were concerned about whether the patient would die and the amount of residual scarring and disfiguration they could expect.

In the acute phase, when patients were resuscitated to the point that they were conscious and could verbalize their feelings, the social worker spent time talking with them about the guilt that many of them felt about their burn injury. She also attempted to relieve them of their anxieties and fears about death or prolonged incapacitation. It was in this phase that patients faced weeks of painful procedures associated with their recovery and the social worker employed relaxation therapy on a few patients to assist them in enduring the pain.

During the weekly team conferences, she was the advocate for the families and tried also to sensitize the other staff members to the patient's socio-emotional needs and problems. Surgeons and nurses tended to look to her for information about how each patient's family was coming to terms with their ordeal and her assessment as to the family's ability to understand and comply with the medical procedures they would become involved in upon the patient's release from the hospital. In this capacity, the social worker was required to gauge the family's emotional readiness and preparedness to care for the patient in the home.

Also, during the acute phase she attempted to support the families in various ways, by periodic assessments of the patient's progress, and by assuring families that the painful procedures being endured by their loved ones were necessary, unavoidable and in the patient's best interest.

Finally, in the rehabilitative phase the social worker was instrumental in securing the going-home arrangements for patients. Since many patients are required post-hospital rehabilitation, it was up to the social worker to put the patient in touch with a variety of community agencies, e.g., Department of Vocational Rehabilitation, that would further assist patients in normalizing their life situations. After patients were released to their homes, they were required to return monthly to the hospital for out-patient examination of their wounds and range of motion. On these "clinic" days, as they were referred to, the social worker visited with each patient and accompanying family inquiring about their problems and concerns in a life now lived outside the burn unit.

Conclusion

In concluding this chapter, I want to summarize briefly a few of the issues raised here and in the Introduction. As I highlight some of the important features of the burn care setting, I will be anticipating what will follow in later chapters, where I hope to deal in much greater detail with some of the ideas being set out here.

We began with the setting: two hospital wards in isolation (in several senses of that term) where critically burned patients were brought for treatment. The burn units themselves were unique in that they functioned both as critical care units and as places of rehabilitation. The staff on the units brought to the setting a perspective of what their work was about, and what they should be doing, to and for whom. Each perspective was unique to that occupation and was neither fully shared nor understood by the other levels of staff. For example, nurses saw their role and responsibilities toward patients from their own perspective as nurses which was, in part, shaped by their special training and the ways "nursing care" was organizationally defined and dictated by senior nurses on the units. As in any medical profession, there were certain problematic aspects of working with the burned that had to be dealt with by the nurses themselves. We looked at one of these problems briefly and that was the part of the nurse's role that required them to cause or inflict pain. While the nurse must work with the team he/she could never completely escape the fact that some of their role demands could only be worked out with other nurses as a colleague-group. Their ways of coming to terms with these problems constituted their "world" and, in turn, determined the way they defined their obligations toward the team.

Again, using nurses as our example, and setting the stage for more detailed analysis later in this book, we can raise some other points of interest about work in a burn care unit. Nurses carried out their daily routines within a context of expectations about the patient's progress toward recovery. These progress expectations, or trajectories, shaped and influenced many of the ways nursing work was conducted. (This was also true of surgeons and therapists.) As nurses put together recovery trajectories for patients it not only guided their work, but also this process was a way of coming to terms for nurses as they began to develop hopes and expectations for a patient's eventual recovery. However, the nursing trajectories were defined on the basis of incomplete information. That is, nurses never fully understood each patient's condition (due, in part, to training limitations), and therefore depended upon other members of the team to fill in the bits and pieces of information about each patient so that trajectories could be modified, updated, etc. This process pulled the nurse into the team matrix and assured his/her continued participation as only other team members had the missing pieces vital to constructing the trajectories. For example, a surgeon could inform a nurse how well a grafting procedure went during surgery; an occupational therapist could give the nurse a good idea of how long a patient would require a particular splint.

While I have concentrated here on the nurse's need for information, in fact, other members of the team developed their own recovery trajectories, and they too relied on others for information to structure their expectations. What made this whole process of information seeking and giving so interesting was that no single level of staff felt they were getting all the information they deserved and perhaps even more importantly, there was a tendency for one level of staff, e.g., surgeons, to make their trajectory ascendant, that is, to get the rest of the team to agree that their recovery trajectory was the most accurate or appropriate. Thus, what I often saw at team conferences was an attempt to arrive at a recovery trajectory for a patient that all team members felt comfortable with or good about. This was not always possible and sometimes while things appeared mutually agreeable in team conferences, afterwards there was often a good deal of grumbling to the effect, "I don't care what the residents' think, Bob is just not ready to go home yet!"

Of course, there was the question of power here, not all team members were equal in the hierarchical structure of the hospital, and it was possible, for example, that the surgeon's trajectory could be dictated to the rest of the team. But, such moves tended to negate the whole idea of team work and would quickly alienate other levels of staff. Physicians were constrained by their need for the good will and support of nurses and therapists, and even more importantly, by their need for information about patients that only nurses and therapists could give! Thus, the term that best captured team relations as it applied to creating recovery trajectories was "negotiation." This refers to a process of give and take among staff positions on the team that permitted them to arrive at some agreeable or common definition of the situation. This give and take among staff proved necessary to maintain some semblance of a common front on those all to frequent occasions when some member of a family would corner a nurse or a resident and ask, "Will Dad be able to come home next week?"

These are the issues that will be the object of our focus in the chapters on dying and recovery trajectories. Before we look at this material and the other features of staff work, however, we must look at the patient experience and that of his/her family, if we are to understand better the problematic nature of caring for the burned.

Chapter Three

PATIENTS AND FAMILIES

THERE were four of us that afternoon in the T.V. lounge, myself and three patients. It was raining hard outside and we could see it splash and beat against the windows of the room. The skies were dark and dreary, but the lounge was well lit, and the large color television set, perched in one corner, had captured our attention now for nearly an hour. There were two large comfortable leather couches in the room, arranged at right angles to each other facing the television. I was sitting next to Ned on one of the couches and Phil and Gary were sitting on the other. The three of them were copiously wrapped in thick white dressings that covered them virtually from head to toe. They would be quite a sight to a stranger, but I was used to it by now. Ned was in his late thirties, medium height and build, he was out-going, relaxed and the most talkative of the three. He had been burned at work while repairing a forge and sustained 40 percent partial and full-thickness burns to his face, neck, arms and chest. He was now in his third week post-burn. Phil was in his middle twenties, a stockily-built, muscular farmer from the southern region of the state. He was quiet and stoic but enjoyed the company in the lounge. His burned covered over 50 percent of his body with his hands suffering the worst damage. It had been over a month now since his tractor caught fire early one morning while he was plowing. He laid in the field for an hour until his father discovered him, but before the morning was over he was admitted to the burn unit. Both hands were covered with grafts to replace the skin he had lost from the fire. Gary had been burned when the gasoline he

56

was using to prime the carburetor on his car exploded in his face. He was burned on nearly 45 percent of his body, mostly partial and full thickness to his face, neck and arms. Gary was tall and athletic, but very shy and withdrawn. In his early twenties, he was the only one of the three men who wasn't married. Normally, he preferred to stay in his room, but Sandi, the occupational therapist, had talked him into sitting in the lounge for awhile, after his exercises.

Each of these three men had undergone at least one surgical grafting procedure and there would be several more to follow. At this point in their recovery, however, they were well enough to be out of bed for an hour or two each day. In addition to their dressings, each of them wore splints over their burned arms, positioned at right angles from their torsos to prevent contractures, so that they had the appearance of white crucified mummies, though most of their faces were visible. They sat gingerly and uncomfortably on the edges of the couches as their donor sites (their own skin used for grafts) had been taken from their thighs and backs and these wounds were now very sore and sensitive when sat upon or leaned against. Phil and Gary used several large foam pillows as cushions for their backs and to rest their arm splints on.

We had been talking on and off as we watched an early afternoon soap opera. Visiting hours were over, and the faces of my three companions gave the impression that they were getting tired and increasingly uncomfortable. In fact, Phil had remarked that he would feel better when he got back to bed and could take a nap. However, we were soon joined by Betty, the unit's social worker, who briskly entered the lounge pushing a large movie projector console. "How would you guys like to see a movie this afternoon? Ned, it's that film I was telling you about. What do you think — are you up for it?" No one offered any objections and I volunteered to go down the hall to find the screen. Within a few minutes, everything was set to go, and Maureeen and Vicki, two of the nurses on duty, decided to watch the film with us. They stood in the rear of the room leaning against a counter running along the wall. Vicki turned out the lights and the movie began.

The film lasted about twenty minutes and was entitled, "He Restoreth My Soul." This was a true story about a gospel and revival minister who was severely burned in a crash of his private plane.

The film depicted the minister reliving the accident, his narrow escape from death, the many months of hospitalization and surgeries, and his subsequent recovery from his burn injuries. Toward the end of the film, the minister recounted how God had tested his faith and though there were many times in the hospital when he had profound doubts concerning his future, his faith was now stronger than ever. This man was facially disfigured from his burns and he described how his belief in God and the support and devotion of his wife helped him accept his stigma. As the film concluded, we saw the minister learning to live with his new appearance as he visited hospitals and burn centers singing for and bringing his message of faith to other victims of disabling accidents. The film was very emotional, but admittedly powerful and somewhat compelling.

When the movie was over Betty found the lights and propped herself upon the edge of a table facing the four of us on the two couches. After a few moments pause she asked, "Well, what did you guys think of that? Any reactions?" There was a period of silence as eyes became accustomed to the light and as each person felt the emotion of the film. Betty looked directly at Ned, "Ned, how do you feel about this film?" He looked up at her and said quietly, "Well, I guess it shows that you just can't give up. No matter how bad things are you keep on going." Betty responded, "O.K. — Phil, how about you?" Phil somewhat awkwardly replied, "When you see other fellars burned worse than you — you don't feel so bad. It's only human to worry about your face. Ned's face here . . . well, it isn't nearly as bad as the guy in that film." Betty nodded silently as Maureeen and Vicki slipped almost unnoticed from the room and disappeared down the hall. There was a long pause as Betty looked in Ned's direction to see if he would respond. Gradually he faced her and said through his swollen lips, "You know Betty, I can accept what I might look like, but I'm worried what my children will think of me. I just don't know what my kids will think — especially my daughter. She's so young . . . and I'm worried about her."

The dialogue continued for a few more minutes, as Betty encouraged each of the three to talk about their feelings. Eventually though, all three became increasingly silent and weary and Betty, sensing that they had enough, began rewinding the film. "We'll have a chance to talk more about this tomorrow if you guys want to." Phil,

Gary and Ned slowly and stiffly began to lift themselves off the couches and soon made their way haltingly back to their rooms. In the burn unit, no patient ever moved quickly.

During a year's time, Betty showed several films to the patients and their families with a discussion following. Usually the movies depicted someone adjusting to a disabling injury and the many triumphs and setbacks along their long road to recovery.

I used the above event to introduce this Chapter on patients and families because it illustrates some of the problems faced by those acutely burned and how they are often made to come to terms. These movies were certainly not the sole therapeutic function of the burn unit social worker, and, it might not be a practice used on other American burn units. But during these observations they were shown and served several social functions in the recovery of burned patients. In analyzing these functions, I hope to give the reader a better understandig of the life and situation of the patient in an adult burn unit.

Most, if not all of the films shown, were inspirational stories of individuals who had recovered and returned to a normal life after a severe burn. For patients in the burn unit such films extended the groups of "others like me" to persons outside the immediate context of the hospital. It gave them a point of comparison of their own situation and condition beyond their fellow patients and made them aware of others in different times and places who were also burned and recovered. Such comparisons allowed each patient to see him/herself relative to others "in the same boat," some of whom were more severely burned. In seeing other victims on film who were sometimes worse off than they, each patient participated in a process known as relative deprivation. They could say to themselves, "as bad as I might think I look, at least my face isn't burned like the woman in the film." This relative deprivation process was a viable and frequently employed coping device for burned patients.

Moreover, such films depicted individuals who were not only burned, but who survived and learned to cope, live and find some measure of happiness and fulfillment. Granted that such messages were highly charged emotionally, nonetheless, patients seemed to find these themes a source of inspiration and usually looked forward to their being shown.

Since burn patients were concerned with their progress toward recovery and rehabilitation, they looked for any occasions to get benchmarks or progress points to see how they were doing or what lay ahead for them. Several of the films did exactly that; in the space of a thirty minute film patients could see an entire recovery trajectory from the moment of the accident through the patient's return home. They could see the various phases of recovery, surgical procedures, healing of scars, etc., layed out in the space of a few minutes. For patients in the second and third month of hospitalization, who were losing track of time and thinking they might never be well enough to go home, these encapsulated recovery trajectories helped to convince them that their time would come too.

Finally, such films were consistent with the burn unit sentimental order; that is, the values, ideals and goals that were shared by the medical, nursing and therapy staffs and permeated their work. The films portrayed burn victims coming to terms with their injuries, cooperating with staff in their recoveries, learning to take hope in the face of setbacks, living with scars and disfigurements, and in the final analysis, affirming life and seeing it was worth the effort. The showing of these films, attended by staff and patients alike, brought them together to symbolically play out the drama of patient recovery on the burn unit. Not that all the patients in this phase of their recovery held these values, as indeed, several did not. There were those patients during the acute stage who were very discouraged, resentful toward the staff, fearful of their disfigurements and profoundly questioning whether life was really worth the daily agony and pain they had to endure. But the films forced them to at least implicitly acknowledge the life affirming values that were part of the moral universe of the medical and nursing staffs. In this sense, the movies reinforced what nurses and therapists had been telling patients all along: "You see, you can do it. It *will* be worthwhile for you just like that minister in the film."

While no patient's attitudes and values were deeply affected or profoundly altered by the movies, nonetheless, several patients admitted to me that they were impressed by the themes and willing to reassess their situations.

To Be Burned

A burn injury is a life-interrupting event. One researcher described it as an accident involving about thirty seconds of terror followed by years of suffering. While several studies show that the majority of burn victims, especially children, make satisfactory social and psychological adjustments after their hospital stays, most of these studies are based on questionnaire and interview data gathered when patients returned for clinic visits in the year or so following release from the hospital. We have little empirical data about the daily lives of burn patients upon their return to society and the fact that patient self-help and support groups are beginning to flourish would indicate that there is a definite suffering component for burn victims that continues long after the hospital experience. In fact, recently some experts have been lead to ask: When is the burn injury healed?

Each burn patient lived out a life and biography on the unit and this was true whether the patient was hospitalized for three weeks or three months. The length of hospital stay shaped only the degree of the biographical career not the kind. In a sense, all burn victims faced the same career contingencies as patients, only some faced them over a longer period of time. A burn injury occured like all accidents when a person least expected it. Within a few moments their lives were wrenched from all that was for them normal and commonplace and familiar to the world of the ambulance, helicopter, emergency room and burn unit; a world that was often unfamiliar, strange and terrifying. It was an event fraught with considerable physical pain, physiological trauma and insult, and psychological anxiety. It was a life-interrupting injury that assaulted the self-hood and taken-for-granted realities of each victim.

Once a patient was admitted to the burn unit their significant others quickly became the nurses, surgeons, therapists and social workers charged with their care. Almost immediately their spouses, parents, children and relatives receded into the background of their reality, appearing only at scheduled and regulated intervals and playing roles defined by the rules and regulations of the burn unit. Their familiar environments of home, neighborhood, playground and work place were abruptly replaced by the hospital room, the Hubbard tank, doctors' rounds and surgery suites. In a span of a few weeks or several months, each patient carved out a career as a burn patient which included a new sense of self and identity; of who they are and what they will become; that was in several ways different from who and what they were before they were burned.

There were, of course, pre-burn personalities and experiences that shaped in part how each patient lived on the unit, e.g., their preferences, prejudices, strengths, and weaknesses that made every individual unique. But the setting of the burn unit itself as a social world of rules, values, ideals, roles and statuses also influenced to a considerable degree the kind of life that each patient would lead. Ultimately every patient, in some manner or another, had to come to terms with the demands and expectations of a variety of medical "others": nurses, therapists, etc., who expected the patient to act in certain kinds of ways and to be certain kinds of people. To the degree that each patient learned to accept and accommodate to these new styles of action and being they gradually came to embrace a new dimension of self.

During the year 1982, the adult unit treated 115 patients, the majority of whom were males and their average age was forty-one years. While no systematic analysis of their social class background was conducted, it appeared that the majority came from working class origins and lower-middle and lower classes. Only a very few patients had professional occupations or college educations. Many had not completed high school. A good number of the male patients were injured in industrial accidents and their hospital bills were covered by Workman's Compensation, however, an equal number of men were marginally employed and had little or no insurance coverage. While all the adult patients were acutely burned, their total body surface area burn ranged from around 15 percent to as high as 95 percent. Most of the adults were injured as a result of flame burns, but there were several patients admitted for electrical burns and a few chemical injuries. Their average length of hospitalization was twenty-two days though several patients were hospitalized for over three months.

The children's unit treated 65 patients in 1982, the majority of which were scald burns. While many of these were the result of accidents, such as children pulling coffee pots over on them, there was a significant number of cases of suspected child abuse or neglect.

More will be said about this later.

There seemed to be an equal number of male and female children burned, the male/female ratio was not as skewed as in the case with adults. Many, if not most, of the children were in the toddler-age groups from about one and a half years to around four years old. Most of the children were not as massively burned as the adults because children cannot survive as large a burn and will die before reaching the hospital. However, a smaller body surface area burn such as 15 percent in a child would be a much more significant injury for them, especially if there was full thickness involvement.

The majority of the children studied here came from the lower socio-economic classes and many were from single-parent households, especially female-head-of-family. These parents rarely had medical insurance and were likely to be receiving food stamps, Aid to Dependent Children and Medicaid. Several parents of burned children were poverty stricken in an almost absolute sense, in that they often had no food to eat nor place to stay while visiting their hospitalized children. Some parents were completely dependent on the burn unit staff to arrange food vouchers for them and sleeping rooms in the local Ronald McDonald's House if available. It was usual, on many nights, for parents to sleep in the hospital rooms with their children, saving the expense of a room and bringing an added measure of security for the children.

For the most part, children did not have as long a stay in the hospital as adults since they were not burned as badly and they tended to heal more quickly and recover physical function. However, several children during the course of the study, did remain on the unit for several months.

In describing the social experiences of burn patients it is not easy to treat the experiences of children and adults as the same. They were not. Adults were much more concerned with their body image, their capacity to endure pain, the interruption in their normal statuses and roles, and what the burn injury meant for their future in terms of their work, community and family life. In short, adults were much more psychologically anxious than were the burned children. Nonetheless, I will attempt to describe some of the more universal experiences of burn patients, recognizing that how these experiences are dealt with and the degree to which they are problematic will vary between children and adults. My purpose in what is to follow is to give the reader a better understanding of the hospital ordeal of patients and then in subsequent chapters, describe how medical, nursing and therapy staffs organize their work, in part, to address these recovery problems. I am now trying to see these problems from the patient's point of view, in later chapters, I will attempt to analyze them from the point of view of staff.

The research literature on the recovery of burn patients agrees that there are definite phases or stages that demarcate the recovery periods. In Chapter Two we labeled these stages: Emergent, Acute and Rehabilitative. Each of the stages brings a different set of problems for the burn patient to adapt to and cope with, though clearly as I hope to show, the Acute phase takes the patient into the closest social relationship with the staff and their requirements for compliance and cooperation.

During the Emergent phase which could last from a few days to, in some cases, several weeks, patients experienced a general psychological confusion, disorientation, dreamlike trances and nightmares. The majority of the disorientation was due to the physiological trauma and shock of the burn injury itself which grossly upset the patient's physical equilibrium causing electrolyte imbalances, for example, which produced a kind of delirium. Patients in the first several days were given pain medications strong enough to induce sleep and numbness so that their other physical injuries could be attended to. In this earliest phase, patients drifted in and out of consciousness and often were not sure what was real and what was dream. Many patients received intensive care in this period; they were connected to ventilators and heart monitors, and received large amounts of fluids through several intravenous lines. All of these strange procedures added to the patient's sense of disorientation and confusion and increased their feelings of helplessness.

Several patients admitted to having night and daymares in which they relived their accidents and could see and feel themselves being burned. Their families often became apprehensive during this period as they worried that the disorientation and confusion might be permanent or indicative of a brain injury. Families were further anxious when patients seemed alienated and estranged from them during their bouts of confusion.

For most patients the emergent phase tended to diminish when they were resuscitated and their bodies recovered from the shock and began to function more normally. This was usually signalled by patients being taken off ventilators and heart monitors; the discontinuing of intravenous fluids and the encouragement of patient ambulation. Interestingly, most patients did not recall much of what happened to them during the Emergent phase. They often appeared amused when their families reminded them of their incoherent babbling and disoriented behaviors.

In the Acute phase, patients were now conscious, usually ambulatory, aware of their condiditons and much more physically, mentally, and emotionally involved in their recovery. As a result, however, they faced a different set of social and psychological problems. Many patients feared they would die from their injuries and needed constant assurances fom staff that they would not. These fears were not entirely unfounded, since not only did they feel very sick and weak; they were in considerable pain. Also, as they became more aware of other patients with them in the burn unit, they occasionally learned of the deaths of fellow patients just down the hall.

The forced dependency troubled a good number of patients who were accustomed to taking care of themselves. Prolonged periods of immobilization through loss of use of arms, hands and legs meant that patients were now almost completely dependent on others for help with their meals, walking, shaving and the ever present and dreaded bed pan.

During the Acute phase patients became aware for the first time of some of the implications of their burn injury. They slowly began to realize that they might not fully regain use of their arms and hands; that they might be permanently scarred and even facially disfigured. Many patients expressed at this point the threats to their identities, personal autonomy and competence as men and women, husbands and wives and workers.

As a result of these fears and anxieties some patients tended to withdraw increasingly from the outside world; a world that they saw all the more threatening, as they became gradually immersed in the world of the burned. Fearing for their competency and identity in the outside world, they began to look for their comfort and security in the burn unit itself. As one recovered burn patient expressed it,

"In the burn unit, it's O.K. to be burned. Everyone accepts you and the way you look. You aren't different in here!"

From the point of view of staff then there were expected periods of regression, depression, denial and withdrawal. These were treated by staff as almost taken-for-granted psychological states that virtually all patients would go through.

It was in the Acute phase that patients coming to terms was most pronounced. For it was at this point that patients experienced the greatest threat to their sense of survival, identity and future and at the same time had to meet the demands of the setting with respect to their recovery. In other words, while they were very anxious about what kinds of persons they now were and would come to be, patients were equally concerned with their capacity to endure the many painful and debilitating procedures and routines that attended their recovery. It was at this juncture that patients began to doubt both their social psychological futures and their present physical abilities. One burn patient, amiddle-aged man with a 60 percent full thickness burn to his neck, arms, legs and chest, and whose recovery had many physical and emotional setbacks, told me one morning after another sleepless night due to his pain, "You know Jim, even if I get through this and can go home — I just don't know whether it will be worth it! You just have no idea how painful this is for me!"

Patients came to terms ina variety of ways and my discussion here will be by no means complete. An entire book could be written about how patients recover from burns and the emphasis in this study is on the staff, but a brief discussion of the patient experience is included here to get a better understanding of how staff responded to this, and how the activities of the staff in turn shape the patient experience.

Some patients embraced rather individualistic devices for support in helping them cope. These persons renewed certain religious commitments if dormant, or heightened still further the religiosity that was already dominant in their lives. Patients took to reading the Bible, looked forward to visits from the chaplain and asked for more attention from their church ministers.They sought a religious strength to help them endure the physical demands now placed upon them and a religious interpretation of why this accident happened to them and of what the meaning of these experiences might be. Still other patients were given inspirational tapes to listen to by members of their family. Such tapes contained inspiring messages of triumph in face of adversity that were usually highly individualistic in orientation and encouraged listeners to look to themselves for strength and the will to succeed. These tapes were often made by successful businessmen and sales personnel.

More often patient looked to the staff or encouragement and support. This was especially the case with adults whose contact with their family was limited to only a few hours per day. This is not to say that the family was not a supportive network for patients, but we'll look more closely at this later in the chapter when we examine how families responded to the hospital experience. The nursing and therapy staff encouraged patients to regard them as a supportive group, by quickly getting on a first name basis and friendly terms with each patient. For adults to the degree that family contact became increasingly limited, much more of their emotion was invested in the nurses and therapists. During the acute phase particularly, nurses and therapists were no longer persons who merely changed their dressings and lead them through their exercises, they were persons who became emotional objects for patients. These emotions ran the gamut from an intense liking, respect, admiration and desire to be close to staff; to the opposite extreme of dislike and sometimes downright hatred. The latter though was rare, most patients, while they developed preferences for some nurses and therapists, nonetheless grew emotionally attached to most of them.

Patients looked forward to seeing certain nurses and to having them assigned to their case for a particular shift. Often patients confided a good deal of their personal feelings, fears, anxieties and prejudices to theirnurses and therapists. A physical therapist, Myra, had been serving another department for about three months when she returned to be burn unit to begin another rotation. She looked into the T.V. lounge on her way to the tank room and spotted Andy, apatient who was in for reconstructive surgery, and who had been a patient of Myra's during the previous summer on his first admission. Myra greeted him, "Hi Andy — what are you doing here?" Andy, "Well, hi Myra! They're working on my flap." "How long will you be in for?" "Oh, a week or two I guess." "Well you look real good and I've missed seeing you." Andy responded, "Thanks, your hair is a lot shorter isn't it? I almost didn't recognize you at first." Myra, "Yes, I'm wearing it shorter now. John and I went to Miami last month for vacation and it was so hot I got it all cut off."

As a result of these emotional attachments to nurses and therapists, patients looked to them not only for support and encouragement in dealing with pain, but also to affirm their identities as worthwhile persons. While their families and relatives were still important to them, it was the nurses and therapists who accepted them totally in their disfigured and mutilated state. Families might and most did come to accept the altered and disfigured appearance of the patient, but usually this took time and some families had difficulty dealing with this issue. For the patients though, nurses, physicians and therapists were a constant, they were never troubled by a patient's appearance. Burned skin that was healing might still look gross and ugly to a patient's friends and family but would draw raves and compliments from the staff! These patients learned from the nurses that they were indeed "looking good."

I'm not overlooking the fact that some patients did resent many of the painful procedures inflicted upon them by staff who were relentless in pushing patients to adhere to exercise schedules, calorie intake and other painful routines. Some patients did develop hostile attitudes toward staff over these issues, but their hostility and resentment was always tempered by their need for the total acceptance that staff showed for their identities as burned people. While the staff might push, berate, chastize, and otherwise make the patient miserable in a physical sense; they were always depended upon by patients to affirm their identity as normal and acceptable people despite their burns.

Ultimately each burn patient faced his/her ordeal alone, but their were occasions for group support that each person got from fellow burn patients. Again this was particularly the case in the acute phase when patients were able to visit with other patients in the lounge. In these sessions each patient would compare his/her progress of wound recovery, pain experiences and problems with coping with others in the same boat. Here those patients more deeply into the recovery trajectory would socialize the less experienced and tell them what they could expect, what was ahead of them and how they might deal with it when it was upon them. The more recently arrived patients looked to the "oldtimers" for progress benchmarks, when they could expect to be grafted; when certain pains would lessen or grow worse; and whether the ugliness of some wounds might begin to disappear. They also learned which nurses and therpists were more gentle in their techniques, more likely to grant special privileges, or were more lenient and liberal in terms of pain medications. It was with respect to pain and its implications that concerned most patients and here "pain talk" and experiences formed the stuff of conversations among patients in the lounge. In fact it seemed at times that patients talked about little else. While normally one would expect that when a group of young males were together the topic of conversation would be centered around cars, excitement, sports or relations with women; such was not the case with young males acutely burned, as the next description illustrates.

One afteroon several patients were talking in the T.V. lounge and the topic was pain. Eric, William, Tom and Bob were all in their late teens and early 20's and with the exception of Tom, all three had been in the burn unit for several weeks. Since Tom had been hospitalized for only a few days, the others were telling him about the future of his pain experiences. Tom had a 15 percent second and third degree grease burn to his arm and shoulder which happened in an accident at work. Tom was mildly boasting that so far his pain wasn't too bad. Eric chided him, "Well . . . I tell ya. That's just the way I felt for the first few days. I felt pretty good myself. And I was braggin — just like you Tom. Well . . . I sure as hell ate my words. All of a sudden it hit me . . . Jesus, it was like I was on fire all over again. God — it just wouldn't stop. Tom, you just wait till they graft you and you get those donor sites. Then you'll know what pain is!"

It was during this acute period that pain became the most difficult ordeal for patients to overcome. Hardly anything that was done to them or for them was not painful. Burn patients were confronted with two temporal aspects of their pain that tested their endurance. In the short run temporally there was the daily pain associated with dressing changes and deridement in which loose dead skin was removed and topical dressings applied to new, raw, and sensitive skin underneath. Many patients found these topical creams to have a burning sensation. Daily exercising of burned limbs which have stiffened and contracted was also painful. And finally, the enforced immobilization of burned limbs in splints, left patients laying for hours in very uncomfortable positions. The other temporal dimension had to do with a longer span of time measured in days and weeks in which as newly regenerated skin buds emerged to replace the burned skin, nerve endings became exposed and pain sensations increased dramatically. As skin began to heal some patients found their pain increased to the point that they began to lose all their tolerance. Accompanying the new skin formation many patients reported itching sensations almost equal in discomfort to the pain itself.

As we shall examine in Chapter four, the burn unit staff tried a variety of pharmacological, psychological and social measures to help patients control their pain behaviors and responses, none of which were totally adequate from the viewpoints of both patients and staff. Research has shown, and my study tends to corroborate, that anxiety can potentiate pain and vice versa. This was especially so in the daily pain experiences of patients who upon awakening each morning began to anticipate what was in store for them in the hours to come. Patients I observed and interviewed, as well as those patients who have written first person accounts of their experiences as burn victims, report the dreaded anxieties of waiting for their turn in the tank room, the ominous sounds of the cart coming down the hall toward their room, the voices of nurses and therapists outside their door signaling that their time had come. As patient anxieties built up concerning how their dressing changes would go that particular day, so too would their pain increase. In this sense, the more worried patients became the more their pain sensations heightened. As the pain on any particular day was especially severe or intolerable the more patient's anxieties increased about the pain that would follow later in the day during exercises or in the evening's dressing change. Thus a vicious cycle was created and presented both staff and patients with an acute coping problem.

While both adult men and women seemed to have similar pain thresholds and even tolerances, males were much more bothered by their pain experiences and consequent pain expressions and behaviors. Several male patients were quite apologetic when they would scream out in pain and appeared embarrassed for themselves later in their interactions with nursing and therapy staffs. Not only were they apologetic, but males tended to find excuses for those occasions when they were particularly vocally expressive in their pain or caused nurses and therapists a difficult time during a dressing change because of their pain responses or behaivors. These patients blamed such occasions on lack of sleep, fears of impending surgery or arguments with wives or girl friends. One male patient asked me repeatedly whether I thought he was being a baby or more bothered by pain than the other men on the unit. He was a muscular, husky-built farmer, and quite disturbed that his pain tolerance was so low and how this seemed to reflect on his sense of manliness.

There are no easy answers as to why males were so bothered by their pain and expressiveness. Possibly males were burned worse or they might have been handled differently than women by the staff during painful procedures. However, observations really didn't confirm this, and I'm lead to believe part of the explanation lies in the socio-cultural values that surround maleness in our society. American males, and particularly working and lower class males are socialized into a pattern of toughness, aggressiveness and independence. Males are expected to rigidly control their emotions and avoid giving in to their feelings. Among working class males this macho image is pronounced as males are required to be brave, strong, virile and virtually impervious to pain.

Many males in this study admitted in part to some of these values in that they boasted that previous accidents and injuries of which they had many never produced the kind of pain they experienced from the burn. In fact, I never talked to a single adult male patient who didn't make it a point to tell me that the burn pain was absolutely the worst they ever felt. Yet, they were continually bothered and upset that such pain caused them to cry or yell or scream! Thus, the burn experience was exceedingly difficult for males to tolerate as the ability to express their pain sensations was so contrary to their patterns of socialization.

Children tolerated pain much better than did the adults and were given less pain medication and sedatives by the staff. In part, this was due to the fact that the children weren't burned as badly, but also it had to do with the medical and nursing staff beliefs that children don't experience pain as intensively as do adults. Such attitudes are substantiated in the research literature which finds that children handle burn pain better and are more easily distracted. The fact that children can be distracted from their thinking about pain could mean that they build up fewer anticipatory anxieties which serves to lessen the amount of pain experienced. This could have been the case but my observations show the problem was more complicated.

On the children's unit, parents and family were very present to the patients due to the liberalized visitation policy that permitted virtually unlimited visiting. Children could have been far less anxious not only about their pain experiences, but about the total hospital experience because of the frequent and in some cases constant presence of their parents and relatives. Moreover, because of developmental differences between toddlers and adults, children might have been less likely to recall and anticipate all that was happening to them. However, many children did know what a trip to get their "bath" meant and would start crying when the nurses, wearing masks and gloves, started walking in their direction. Children rarely attempted to control their pain expressions and behaviors during their tubbings as did adults. They shrieked, screamed, kicked and flailed thoughout the dressing changes and such vocalizations could be heard from far away. However, once the tubbing was over, the children quickly returned to their play activities as if nothing had happened. Perhaps this "letting go" provided children with a release of emotion and affect which made the pain experiences more tolerable and bearable, whereas the adults attempts to control their responses because of cultural mandates and setting requirements and decorum served to intensify their feelings of being in pain. Even when adults did let go and vocalize their pain, it often seemed to make them feel worse for "giving in" and, as I have said earlier, they were often quick to apologize for having lost control.

When we attempt to analyze children's pain responses and sensations, however, we need to be very cautious because at the toddler level of development children either cannot or do not give accurate and sophisticated accounts of their pain experiences. Thus, while staff assumed that children had less pain and tolerate it better than adults, such assumptions might not have any physiological basis at all, and could be due to childrn's developmental inabilities to clearly articulate what their pain means and just how debilitating they might have found it to be.

Patient Progress

One morning in the tank room, Ned was lying in the Hubbard tank while Joan, the physical therapist, was gently peeling some of the dead burned tissue from his shoulder. Ned asked her, "I didn't hear what the doctor told me this morning at rounds about whether I was going to get grafted. Did you hear what he said?" Joan answered him, "I didn't hear what your doctor said. I wasn't close enough, Ned." After a few minutes Joan took me aside and said quietly, "During rounds everyone talks to everybody but the patient. No one says anything to them! I guess I don't agree with the team concept if it doesn't include the patient."

Ned, like all burn patients was trying to get a better idea of his fate, of what was in store for him in the days and weeks ahead. A major burn injury takes weeks and even months to heal and in the case of full-thickness or third degree injuries, surgery will be required. If a patient was a large percentage of third degree, several surgeries will be forthcoming usually spaced a few weeks apart. The life of the burn patient then is marked by the ebb and flow of surgical events, but also by the patients physiological ability to fight off infection which can inhibit wound healing. Not all wounds heal at the same rate and much of the healing depends on each individual's physiological capacity to recover.

All patients, but particularly the adults, were concerned about their progress: how their wounds were healing; whether grafts were taking and how closely they were on their timetable of recovery. While in time most patients learned to evaluate their wounds, to look for the signs of new and healing skin, they nevertheless depended mostly on the staff for information about their progress. Thus in the Acute and Rehabilitative stages, patients looked to the staff to gauge their readiness to go home and begin their return to normal life.

Burn unit staff, for their part, imparted varying amounts of prognostic information, muchof it indirect and usually couched in cautionary terms to the effect that while there might be some positive signs, patients must always be prepared for setbacks. Though staff was normally upbeat, and optimistic in their relations with patients they also admonished them that burn injuries take along time to heal. Furthermore, patients were told to never "give up," yet, they should take one day at a time and learn to look for small signs of gradual improvement rather than dramatic breakthroughs.

As you might expect, some patients got frustrated with the staff's constant optimism, particularly in light of the fact that most patients recovered very slowly and recovery signs were measured in weeks rather than days. The following comments by Val, a male patient in his fifth week post burn are a case in point. Val had 20 percent burns to his neck, shoulders and arms which required several surgeries.

"Whenever they (surgeons) look at my grafts they always say, 'that's great! The look real good.' Well, I asked them just what does this mean? 100 percent good or 95 percent good — or what? Is there some part that didn't take so well? All anyone says around here is that everything is good. God . . . everything is so optimistic. But when that is all you hear you begin to get suspicious. Not everything can be that good all the time!"

Patients learned never to fully trust all the prognostic information they received from staff, although they often tended to value the information given by the surgeons more than the nurses and therpists. This is somewhat ironic considering that surgeons gave far less information to patients than did other staff and spent less time communicating with patients in general.

The ability of patients to obtain prognostic information about their condition was related to these variables: their socio-economic and educational status; their aggressiveness in seeking information; and the assertiveness of family and friends. Actually all three of these variables were interrelated.

As stated earlier most of the adult patients were of working class and lower class origins and their educational levels were such that they were not always articulate and able to verbalize easily their needs and feelings with the staff. Many patients were in awe of the surgeons in particular, and the educational and expertise attainments of the burn unit staff in general. Thus many patients had difficulty expressing themselves with staff especially in asking for concrete and accurate assessments of their current state and futures. Staff tended to reinforce those feelings of inadequacy on the part of patients by often assuming that they were not intellectually capable of knowing what was best or able to comprehend the sophisticated physiology involved in wound recovery. I'm not arguing that patients were left totally in the dark about their progress toward recovery, but the information given to them was often indirect, vague and rarely explained fully the the patient's siatisfaction. The following description illustrates this problem of information seeking.

Warren was in his early twenties and had been a patient on the unit for over three weeks. His grafts were healing well and he was anxious to get home but no one was saying much about it to him. He had tried several times to "fish" for information from his nurses about where he stood in terms of going home. Today he tried again. Warren and his nurse Vickie were sitting in the lounge, Vickie was sitting on one of the couches writing her medication charts while periodocially glancing at the soap opera on the television. Warren sat on the other couch watching the television but was restless and smoked one cigarette after another. Both had been silent for several minutes when Warren said causually, "By the way Vickie, do they let you know in advance when you get out of here — or do they just tell you the day before?" Vickie responded without looking up from her chart, "Oh, I'm sure someone will tell you when you're ready. They'll give you a week's notice." Warren didn't question her furhter, he sat there silently alternating his gaze between the television show and Vickie who continued to write busily in her chart. Maureen, another nurse on duty, looked into the lounge to say something to Vickie and Warren got her attention. "Maureen, when am I getting out of here?" Maureen said without hesitation, "Seven to 10 days." And without another word and without looking at Warren she quickly left the room and walked down the hall. Warren looked in her direction and with a puzzled look on his face, shrugged his shoulders, and then turned his attention back to the television.

Patients with professional occupations and high educational attainments were, however, noticeably more able to get fuller and more detailed staff appraisals of their current situations, future surgical plans, and even possible release dates. This was partly due to their aggressiveness in that the better educated patients with higher status occupations were more demanding about their rights to receive information. These patients had a more commanding presence of the burn unit and would voice their displeasure if the information they sought was not forthcoming or presented clearly and accurately for them. Since the staff tended to view such patients as their "equals," they in turn gave them more complete and medically sophisticated assessments because it was assumed that these patients could "handle" it. One such patient was a university professor injured in a laboratory experiment. He sustained severe burns to his face, neck and hands in the explosion. The surgeons treated him deferentially throughout his stay as his status as a scientist warranted full disclosure of all medical procedures and prognosis. However, during the first week or two on the burn unit, this patient was very shy and passive in asking for information. He was no more assertive than the other patients on the unit and occasionally had to be prompted by the nurses to ask the surgeons about things he considered important. The nurses encouraged his boldness with the surgeons since they knew that given his exalted status on the unit the physicians would not hedge or put him off. As a consequence, during the later stages of his hospitalization he was quite talkative and aggressive in dealing with surgeons knowing he could pretty much get his way in most things. Subsequent to his release from the hospital when he would return for clinic appointments to have the surgeons check theprogress of his at-home recovery and make decisions about reconstructive surgery; he was quite prepared to get all the information about his progress he felt he deserved. He would bring to clinic a yellow legal table with a list of questions he wanted the surgeons to answer. Slowly and methodically he would ask each question and then check it off when it was anwered to his satisfaction. This took up to fifteen or twenty minutes and the medical director showed no irritation or impatience at being inconvenienced by the length of this examination. In fact, the conversation took the tone of collegiality rather than the usual hesitant and awkward questioning by a patient of her/his surgeon. The majority of other patients returning to clinic were rarely afforded that much careful attention and communication by the surgeons.

Thus, patients aggressiveness in asking for and even demanding information was related to their occupational and education status. Since few of the patients were highly accomplished in these areas, cases such as the professor's stood out and the deferential manner of their treatment was noticeable even among the staff.

The family of the patient can also advocate on his/her behalf in the quest for detailed prognostic information. This was particularly the situation with children, many of whom were too young to ask the staff about their progress. With children it was the parents and family that needed this information and whether they received it depended in part on how aggressively they sought it. The nursing staff on the children's unit was more open with families than the staff on the adult unit. They welcomed the questions that parents had about their children's condition as that was taken as a sign of parents interest and competency. Since nurses on the children's unit were somewhat eager to involve the parents in the daily care of their children, the inquisitive and interested parent was seen as someone who would be willing to coopeate and get absorbed in the social life of the burn unit. The nursing staff was usually willing to give a good deal of prognostic information in return for the parents continuing involvement.

On the adult unit, families received about the same kind and amount of information as the patients; scattered, vague and somewhat incomplete. However, the families were not in the dependent patient role and thus were a bit more free to pursue the staff for information. In fact, often it was the family that received whatever information that was forthcoming and this was passed on to the patient during visiting hours. In some cases, the family was much more demanding and assertive than the patient and at other times nurses felt the family could handle the information better than the patient and left it to the family to decide how much they would share with them. Patients often saw themselves in partnership with their family in obtaining information about their progress and during visiting hours the conversation would consist of patients and families sharing the bits of data each had received from various sources attempting to put together a coherent mosaic of the patient's recovery trajectory.

Rehabilitative Phase

Toward the end of theAcute phase as the patients' wounds began to heal and they were increasingly able to take care of themselves in activities of daily living, the patients experienced a renewed interest in the outside world. This shift was gradual rather than abrupt and was characterized by ambivalent feelings toward the burn unit and it's staff. On the one hand, most patients felt very good about the care they received, the friendships that were made and their ability to survive the injury. On the other hand, a return of interest in the outside world was acutally a sign of recovery; patients were catching up psychologically with their continuing physical improvement. Patients became anxious to return home, to renew various roles and statuses that they had forfeited for several weeks and months and to tentatively try out their new identities as burned people.

Letting go of the burn unit and it's safe, secure and protected environment was not an easy task for some patients. They often felt secure in the competency manifested by their nurses and therapists. One patient, who was transferred to another ward during the final week of his hospitalization to make room for a more critical patient, returned to the burn unit the day of his release from the hospital. He told two of the burn unit nurses, "Boy . . . I didn't know what good care was until I left here!" Later I asked him about this and he said that on the other ward the nurses had too many patients to take care of and they couldn't give him the individual attention that he needed. Also, since the nurses on the other ward weren't accustomed to working with burns they just didn't have the confidence in taking care of him. He worried during dressing changes, for example, that the nurses wouldn't do them correctly and he would be left uncomfortable or improperly wrapped.

Patients also had difficulty giving up the primary-like relations they had developed with the staff, particularly the nurses and therapists. Many patients felt close emotionally to certain of their therapists and nurses because of the intimacy of that healing environment, thus, giving up the burn unit meant an end to that closeness and intimacy. Granted that much of what the staff did to patients was painful, in the Rehabilitative phase much of that pain was now forgotten as patients focused on their attachments to the staff. This closeness was expressed in several ways. Mark, a nurse on the children's unit was preparing to go home at the end of his shift and while in his street clothes he walked back into the unit saying, "I better say good-by to my girls!" He was referring to the 3 toddler-age patients he had been caring for during the day. On the adult unit one patient recorded a message on a cassette tape the day of his discharge in which he thanked virtually every staff member by name for the care he had been given. This was a highly emotional message, expressing his fondness for everyone, and how much he would miss the staff, and it ended with a very tearful farewell.

During the Rehabilitative phase as the patient prepared both physically and emotionally to return home, this renewed interest in the outside world was occasionally accompanied by feelings of irritability and hostility toward the staff and even family members. Some patients lost their tempers, refused to eat or exercise and began to complain incessantly about pain and itching discomforts. Researchers have argued that this phenomenon is due to the patient's awakening libidinal ties to important persons; that in their desire to return to their familiar settings outside the hospital, there is a kind of emotional flood or cascade of feelings toward important persons, but these feelings or emotions are not always in control. This was the case with several patients who seemed to be testing the strength of the relationships they had built up with staff by pushing the tolerance limits of compliance and cooperation norms. It had also to do, I feel, with the ambivalency of patient's feelings for the burn unit, during the Rehabilitative phase. Such patients were caught in the emotional pushes and pulls of wanting to remain safe, secure, accepted and cared for, yet, anxious to test the waters of the outside world to see for themselves first hand their ability to act with autonomy and competence in their homes and communities. The Rehabilitative phase, the first few days or weeks of preparing to go home, left patients in limbo, with the ambivalent status of persons between identities.

Interestingly, the staff often became upset when patients acted out this ambivalency in an uncooperative, cranky and hostile manner. Nurses, for instance, interpreted these behaviors as a loss of morale, a moving backwards and loss of ground. These patients were accused of not showing proper gratitude toward staff for all they had done for them, and staff began to wonder about the "immaturity" of such patients and their ability to function adequately upon their return home. In the worst of these cases, nurses and therapists expressed sentiments that they were at the end of their ropes with those patients and couldn't wait for them to go home.

During those cases where patients became very difficult to care for there was the curious phenomenon of nurses and therapists "giving up" on a patient who was in an emotional sense having an equally difficult time "letting go." When such patients most needed the encouragement to face a new world and give voice to their emotions they were most likely to be left alone and avoided by the therapists and nurses.

Families

There is an old saying, appropriate in an era of war, to the effect: "They also serve who only sit and wait." Such was the lot of families of burn patients who were expected to be supportive of their loved ones, but who found themselves with a lot of time on their hands and relatively few ways within the hospital to fill it. There was a significant difference, however, between the adult and children's unit in that the adult unit had a restrictive visitors policy and the children's unit a very liberalized one. Families of adults were permitted only 6 hours of daily visitation, from 11:00 a.m. to 2:00 p.m. and from 5:00 p.m. to 8:00 p.m. Only the immediate family could visit the patient, e.g., wives, parents, grandparents, etc., and only two visitors were allowed at a time. On the children's unit, families had unlimited visiting privileges and parents could sleep in the same room with their children. These differences in visitation policies between the two units shaped the experiences of families in important ways. However, there were some modes of adaptation among families in both units that were held in common.

Families in each of the two units formed spontaneous and unplanned support groups for each other. Social relations among families were quickly upgraded as families rapidly got to know each other, compared experiences, helped each other out in daily living, and supported one another in times of crisis. Traditional barriers of class, education, race and age were temporarily suspended as each of the families recognized their common bond and looked toward each other for sources of strength and encouragement. For these families, the crisis of the burn injury was their common denominator.

While the families supported and helped each other through the weeks and months of their ordeals, their central energies, however, were invested in their burned son, daughter, spouse or parent. Usually, and without recognizing it explicitly, the families became the advocate for the burn patient, which was a blending of supportive attitudes and protective tendencies on the patient's behalf. Families held tenaciously to the ideal that they were there to protect the interests of their loved one, alleviating as much of the suffering as they could. In this regard, some families took it upon themselves to cushion the patient from the demands of the burn unit staff. They often confronted the nurses, since they were the most visible, to ask that their family member be given more pain medication, be made more comfortable, or be excused from therapy sessions, or given special privileges to make their odeal more tolerable.

It was in this area that families of burn patients could either upset the sentimental order of the burn unit or act in ways to affirm it. From the point of view of the nursing staff, the behaviors of families could not be taken-for-granted. It could not be merely assumed that families would be conforming, cooperative, and supportive of the regime of burn care that formed the basis of what was done to and for patients. In so far as staff was concerned, families could neither be ignored nor counted on to do what was right. Families were needed for a variety of reasons, including the fact that they were an audience for what the staff was trying to do on patient's behalf. And like all performers, the burn unit staff not only wanted to perform correctly, i.e., to help burn patients recover; they wanted to look good in the process.

Thus, the staff, in leaving little to chance, actively engaged the families in the recovery process. They were given a role to play. For their part, most families, but not all, wanted to be drawn in. They sought a function, a chance to help, an opportunity to contribute to the recovery of their family member. However, the staff engaged the families on their own terms; families were given a role to play and a chance to perform but within a definite structure of rules, regulations, and expectations to which they were obligated to conform. If families wanted to be part of the team, they were expected to adhere to the rules of the game.

The children's unit and the adult unit took different approaches in handling and managing the families of their patients. While both units emphasized cooperation and conformity to the rules and regulations, the adult unit encouraged the families to *support* their patients and the children's unit encouraged a more encompassing *involvement* of the families in the recovery/care of their patients. I will examine first the dynamics of family support and cooperation in the adult unit.

Florence was a nurse on the adult unit evening shift; tall and slender she was in her 20's and had worked on the unit for several years. As she walked into the nurses lounge at the beginning of her shift she said to Sheri, one of the day shift nurses, "God . . . George's family about attacked me just now as I was coming in. They are so damned hyper!" Sheri replied, "Well they're concerned about their dad and I guess if it were mine, I would be too." Florence, "Last night his daughter kept complaining that we weren't explaining everything to them. Well, I got mad and that only made things worse. They told Virginia (Head Nurse) that they didn't want a nurse who was mad at them taking care of their father. So I called the one daughter aside later and told her not to worry — her father would get the best of care." Sheri, "Florence, this is a family that needs to be kept informed about everything. George's oldest daughter is a nurse and I guess she will be the go-between for the family. We just need to let her know everything we're doing and she'll tell the others. They need lots of TLC."

In the above description, taken from field notes, George' family was not too atypical, they were merely more vocal in getting what they wanted and when the burn unit staff learned that one of the daughters was a nurse, they felt that maximum cooperation was possible if that daughter were kept better informed about what was being done to her father. Nurses in the adult unit managed families by trading information that the family wanted and needed about the status of patients in exchange for assurance that the family would: conform to the rules about visitation rights; permit the staff to carry out their work with a minimum of interference; support the patients through encouraging them to comply with demands associated with their recovery. Such a bargain was always implicit and tacitly agreed upon rather than explicitly negotiated. Also, like most bargains, it was rarely totally adhered to by both parties.

Nurses and therpists recognized that patient's families were a ready source of patient encouragement and emotional support. They realized that their own abilities in this area were limited even though patients looked to them for approval and acceptance. In addition, patients were to return to their families in the long run and such a transition was likely to be more smooth if families entered into the supportive matrix during the patients hospital stay. However, nurses also realized that the family was an important vehicle for insuring patient compliance to the recovery program. In fact, this was the implicit meaning of the term support; to provide the patient with the social and psychological motivation to cooperate in her/his recovery treatment. In practical terms this meant motivating the patients to: endure their pain with a minimum of medication, engage in the daily physical exercises; wear their splints properly and consistently; and maintain their daily level of calorie intake. At another level support meant persuading patients to do all of the things willingly and cheerfully!

Family support on the adult unit was often elicited in the weekly meetings between a representative of the nursing staff and the families of patients currently on the unit. These meetings, held in the family waiting room, and announced by posters placed near the waiting room were open to all interested families. The sessions were lead by a burn unit nurse who educated families about burn wound recovery, both its physiological dimensions and its psychological implications. Occasionally, families were treated to slide presentations of techniques in wound care and phases of patient recovery. Also, in these sessions the nurses would explain the meaning and importance of the various procedures used in treating burn patients. It is this aspect that concerns us here. The following is based on field observation of one of these family education sessions.

June, one of the nurses who often led these meetings was instructing a group of families about the importance of splints and why patients must be encouraged to wear them at times specified by the occupational therapist. "I know you feel we push our patients too hard and sometimes what we do looks cruel to you. But I can't emphasize too much how important this rehabilitation function is! You must remember, 'The position of comfort is the position of deformity.' If patients stay in comfortable positions their arms will contract that way and they'll lose their range of motion. Eventually they will need more surgery. So, they need your support in this. It's tough on the patients! It really is . . . and they need you in their fight to keep going. They need help from persons who don't cause them pain." Later in the meeting June encouraged the families to ask the nurses about anything they didn't understand. "I want you to feel free to ask us questions. Even if it looks like we're busy. Just ask us if there is something you don't understand."

Here the implicit bargain is almost made manifest. Nurses ask that the families support the recovery program of the burn unit and in turn the nurses agree to keep them informed. This drawing in process had positive functions and actually served families and staff rather well; it allowed the staff greater control over their work situation in that families were encouraged to be their allies in the recovery process, and families were made to feel an important part of the recovery of their loved ones.

I am reserving my analysis of this involving process among families of burn children until the close of the chapter when I address the importance of family involvement in still greater detail.

In addition to the involvement mechanism with respect to families, there were two other ways in which burn unit staff related to patients' families. One, they kept families informed in varying ways and degrees about the progress of patients. Secondly, staff initially prepared families about the realities of burn injury recovery.

Families of burn victims were often as initially distraught with the circumstances of the burn injury as the patients. They too were thrown suddenly and unpreparedly into the world of the hospital in general and burn units in particular and many families found it a very trying experience. Among their earliest and most pressing concerns was whether or not the patient would live. At first, that seemed most important and sometimes all they would or could ask for. Later, however, they discovered that burn victims could live for several weeks before they died so that any initial optimism had to be tempered with a good deal of caution. Families also learned that patients could be very sick for a long period of time and they would have to search rather constantly for clues as to what kind of progress their family member was making.

Information about patients was given to families at various stages during a patients stay, but staff and families alike expected that when a patient was admitted to the burn unit, some explicit details about chances for survival or recovery expectations would be offered. Often the nurses assumed this role especially if staff anticipated that the patient would recover from the burn injury. The description below shows how these initial assessments were given to families.

Ned was in his late thirties and sustained a 40 percent body surface burn to his face, neck, arms and chest from an explosion in the factory where he worked. His wife, Barb, rode with him in the ambulance to the hospital, but remained in the family waiting room as Ned was wheeled into the burn unit. Virginia, the head nurse, was in the tank room when the surgeons and nurses made their preliminary evaluations of his wounds and other injuries, and later she came into the waiting room looking for Barb. Virginia beckoned for Barb to join her in the hall away from the other families in the room. Looking directly at Barb, Virginia began, "Ned has 40 percent second and third degree burns to his arms and chest. But, he's doing fine and there shouldn't be any problem." Barb asked her, "Do you have any idea how long he will have to stay here?" Virginia answered, "He'll be in here for two months — that's what we told him. It might turn out a little less, but we don't want to get his hopes up. It's better to let him know he'll be here for a long time." Barb, acted a little bewildered, "Do you think he can take that?" Virginia said softly and distinctly, "Well Barb, he's got a lot going for him. He's young and he tolerates pain well." Barb brightened up a little, "Yes . . . Ned's that way. He doesn't complain much. He was awake in the ambulance all the way here! Can I touch him?" Virginia smiled, "Yes, you can. I'll get you some gloves. Now Barb . . . his face is going to swell up and his eyes may swell shut for a few days. But that's normal and nothing to worry about. You're going to need a gown too Barb."

Notice that assurances were initally given that Ned would survive, but also, an indication that his recovery would be a long slow process. Virginia also gave reason for optimism for Ned's recovery in that his age and endurance were positive factors, but implied as well that his ability to accept his pain would be a crucial factor.

When patients were more severely burned than Ned and there was some question among the staff as to whether the patient would survive, it was often up to the surgeons to prepare the family, since it was assumed that families would be more likely to accept the surgeon's word in these matters rather than the nursing staff. Also, nurses felt more comfortable when the surgeons confronted the family if there was any doubt the patient might not make it. Here is an example from field notes.

David was an out-of-work mechanic, forty years old, a heavy drinker and smoker, who sustained 80 percent third degree burns when someone doused him with gasoline and set him on fire. In addition to his burns, he suffered severe smoke inhalation, and was intubated at the scene and placed on a ventilator immediately upon his arrival at the burn unit. He was unconscious thoughout.

Joel was the senior resident on duty the day David was admitted and after examining his wound, he found David's wife Lucy in the hall outside the burn unit and took her into the conference room and asked her to sit down. Lucy was in her thirties, with gray hair and a tired and worn look on her face. She chained smoked while Joel was talking to her. "Your husband has a very serious injury but I think he has a decent chance of making it. If you take a person's age plus the percent of their body burned — that is their probability of dying. David is 40 and he's burned over 80 percent of his body. So you can see what we're up against. Ah . . . so I'd say that he as less than a 50/50 chance of making it. He'll be in the critical stage for several days maybe even weeks. There are different stages a burn patient goes through and I'll let you know how he is doing at each stage. I'll talk to you whenever you want to . . . but I might not have much to say." There was a short pause and Lucy said, "Well, right now I'm worried about the money. David hasn't worked in 7 months. We don't have much laid back in case of an emergency." Joel told her, "You see the social worker, her name is Betty and she'll help you with that. But don't worry — it won't affect the care we give him. We could care less who can pay their bills and who can't. Do you have any other questions?" Lucy paused to put her cigarette out and then looked up at Joel, "Yes, doctor. Who would want to burn my husband like that?" Joel answered her, "I don't know."

Joel talked to Lucy for several more minutes as she thought of further questions about visiting privileges and where she could find lodging, etc. Joel was patient with her and she accepted his trajectory of guarded optimism. Note that while he told her David had less than a 50/50 chance to survive, he did leave room for hope by informing her about a stage process of patient recovery! David never regained consciousness and died three days later of complications associated with his lung injury. Not all the staff agreed with Joel's somewhat optimist stance toward David. Some of the nurses felt he had little chance at all of surviving and that his wife should have been told that. Joel, however, argued that he had prepared Lucy adequately and realistically — giving her the opportunity to calculate that her husband's chances were not great, but also giving her some reason to hope. This was most often the case in that families were rarely told that a situation was hopeless except in those few instances when patients were brought in literally charred to the bone and died within a few hours.

After families were initially prepared for some of the eventualities in recovery and given a tentative prognosis, they were pretty much left to themselves to uncover other pieces of prognostic information as the patient's stay continued. Staff did not routinely inform families about patient progress and this was due in part to their own uncertainty. Burn wounds healed very slowly and progress benchmarks were neither dramatic nor frequent. Patients tended to improve or worsen gradually rather than abruptly and the signs of both conditions were few, subtle and very technical. Nonetheless, families did long for some indications of how well their love ones were doing and how near they might be to going home. They sought such information from all levels of staff, but received most of it from nurses and therapists. Surgeons were much less visible on the unit and when they did appear to examine patients they hurried in and out in a manner that did not encourage families to stop them and ask questions. However, some families did become bold and could be seen scurrying down the hall after the surgeons trying to get their attention and hoping for something in the way of good news.

Nurses were often a go-between for surgeons and families. Surgeons used the nurses to pass information about a patient's condition to the family, giving the nurse the latitude to tell them as little or as much as she/he might choose. Likewise the nursing staff would convey to the surgeons a particular family's concerns about what was going on and the physician's response and evaluation would then be passed on the family by the nurse. On some occasions nurses asked the surgeons directly if they would be willing to speak to a family or spouse especially if the nurses had assured the family that the doctor would indeed talk to them.

There were some situations, however, where a patient's condition warranted a direct talk with the family to apprise them of a significant change in trajectory or to impress upon them the seriousness of the patient's current state. The following, taken from field notes, describes such a situation in which a nurse confronted the family.

June, one of the burn unit nurses was given the responsibility of having a conference with the family of Lonny, a seventeen year old male who was burned severely in an automobile crash. In addition to his burns, Lonny suffered a massive head injury and was unconscious for over 10 days after admission to the burn unit. His family visited him frequently and insisted on spending more time in his room than the nurses felt appropriate given his critical condition. June was to have a talk with the family to impress upon them Lonny's need for more quiet and rest and to convince them of the seriousness of his injury. She told Audry, the head nurse, before she was to meet with the family, "I'm going to begin all my sentences with, 'If he survives . . .' maybe then they'll get the message."

At other times, families would initiate a dialogue with staff in asking directly for progress information. Even surgeons would submit to the encounter and give rather detailed information if they felt that some significant benchmark had been reached. That is to say, if a patient had arrived at a significant point in their recovery it constituted "good news" and in these cases surgeons were quite willing to be the bearer of glad tidings.

I was with Joel, the senior resident, one morning and after the completion of rounds he walked into the family waiting room and stood in front of a young woman, "You wanted to talk with me?" Shirley was in her early twenties and was the fiance of Bobby, who was in his fourth week of hospitalization for second and third degree burns to 90 percent of his body. Shirley said quietly to Joel, "Yes . . . I'd like to know how Bobby's doing." Joel sat down next to her on the couch, "Well . . . he's out of the woods. He will recover — although I'll tell you that those wounds on someone older would have been lethal. Bobby's going to survive because he's so damn ornery!" Shirley smiled and then laughed softly. Joel continued, "He's been the ideal patient. When he gets well he'll have to come back and be a cheerleader for other patients. Now . . . when we start to graft Bobby he'll be over the hump." Shirley, "Will all of his legs need to be grafted?" Joel shook his head slowly, "No — not completely. I think that some of it will heal on its own. But about 50 percent of both legs will need grafts." Shirley, "How soon after that will he be better . . . you know . . . able to go home?" Joel, "It's still going to be many weeks. He's got a long way to go, but he'll make it." Shirley was all smiles and blushed slightly as she thanked him. Joel rose from the couch and started toward the door, but stopped about half-way and turned back to Shirley "The reason I didn't talk to you more was that I didn't have anything to tell you. But now I do." Joel walked back to Shirley, shook her hand and then quickly left the room.

This surgeon, Joel, was no more willing to talk to families than any other resident. In fact, he once told me his technique of sliding along the wall past the family waiting room to the stairwell in such a way that he could dash for the stairs and disappear before families could catch him. He spent nearly ten minutes with Shirley because she had been insistently asking for an audience with him and he eventually had something significant to tell her. Surgeons were much more able to pick and chose their occasions for communicating with families than were the nurses, who were so highly visible to the families that they were faced almost daily with their requests for information. When nurses hedged or spoke only in the most general and/or vague terms, families were often suspicious and resentful feeling that nurses were hiding something or unwilling to give them the attention they deserved. Families were less disturbed with the infrequent communication they had with surgeons, but prized any encounter that had with them and accepted their word for things as absolute.

Family Involvement

Both the adult and children's burn unit attempted to get families involved in the recovery of patients. As we saw, in the adult unit this involvement was limited to engaging families to act cooperatively, and to support patients and staff in the various aspects of the recovery program. However, in the very final days of the Rehabilitative phase, when patients were being prepared to go home, their families were encouraged to get more actively involved in care by learning to do the dressing changes that they would have to assist the patient with upon their return home. Most burn patients were discharged from the unit with some areas of their wounds incompletely healed. These areas would have to be carefully cleansed and dressed twice daily with special medications and gauze wrappings, and on the final days of a patient's stay families were taught these dressing techniques. For many families on the adult unit these practice sessions were their first glimpse of the burn wounds that their loved ones had sustained. This proved to be a trying experience for some families as they confronted for the first time the ugliness of the wounds and their own squeamishness and awkwardness in handling them. Such families were forced very quickly to come to terms with the fact that while the patient was finally returning home, they were bringing with them ugly and disfiguring wounds that would not soon disappear.

Some of the nurses on the adult unit were aware of how difficult this abrupt transition was for families, and began to wonder if they should have been encouraging families to get involved in recovery care sooner and more comprehensively. This could have been accomplished by a more flexible visitation policy and permitting families to assist with dressing changes earlier in the patients recovery. These ideas were discussed by two nurses in the next excerpt from field notes.

Maureen, one of the day shift nurses, and Audry, the head nurse, were having coffee together one morning in the nurses lounge. Maureen had just finished the dressing changes on Alice, a woman in her late fifties who had suffered severe burns to her chest, arms and neck. During the course of several surgical procedures one of her breasts was now nearly gone as it had been burned so deeply. Alice was close to being able to go home and neither she nor her husband had seen her wounds unwrapped. Maureen remarked to Audry, "I just know Alice is going to be bothered by her appearance, Audry. And her husband will be too. She just doesn't have any breast left there at all! When I tell her it (breast) looks good — it's not what she means by looking good. I'm talking about the wound! I just wonder if we should have involved Alice's family sooner in her care . . . so they could be prepared for what her breast is going to look like. What do you think?" Audry, slowly sipping her coffee, "Well — we still have a few days before she's leaving. Maybe we should talk to Betty (social worker) about it tomorrow in team conference." Maureen shook her head in agreement, "You know I'm beginning to question if our policy of keeping the family out of it until the final few days is wrong. Maybe they should be brought in sooner." Audry nodded, "I think we should be creating an atmosphere where patients feel comfortable and more independent to make their own decisions. You know I might favor 24 hour visiting! That would *really* get them involved!"

The issue of the family role in patient recovery on the adult unit was never fully resolved during the research period. Families continued to occupy a rather ambivalent position. On the one hand, they were recognized, informed to varying degrees, prepared for various contingencies, and encouraged to be supportive of the patients. On the other hand, they were often in the dark about much of what was going on in the unit and their presence in the lives of patients was limited to the few hours per day they were allowed to visit. I should add here, however, that the restrictive visitors's policy of this unit was very typical of the practices of the other burn units in the country that I look at.

The children's burn unit by contrast actively sought the involvement of parents and family throughout the recovery process. Such objectives were even included in the nursing charts where nurses listed as objectives in patient care, the involvement of families and methods they would used to bring this about. As discussed earlier, parents were free to visit their children on a 24 hour per day basis. Families were encouraged to feed their children, read to and play with them, and even maintain normal disciplinary practices when appropriate. Parents were also given the opportunity to assist the nurses in the daily tubbings and dressing changes and many parents did. Some had difficulty with this though as wound care tended to upset them both physically and emotionally, and these parents often asked to be excused from this activity until the last days of a child's hospitalization when they could hardly avoid it any longer.

While I have used the term "parents" here when referring to families, I need to point out that it was the female side of families that were engaged in most of these activities: mothers, grandmothers and occasionally aunts. Male participation was limited to visiting in a restrictive sense and many of the children had few male figures present in their lives while on the burn unit.

In the course of my observations there were a significant number of children whose burns were sustained through parental neglect and abuse. Nurses told me that the year 1983 seemed especially rife with cases of child abuse. In these instance, burn unit staff filed a "310" which was a special form denoting suspected neglect or abuse and that would trigger an investigation by the Department of Child Protective Services and the appropriate police jurisdictions. Thus it was not unusual to see detectives visiting the burn unit, taking pictures of the child's wounds for court evidence and interviewing staff to get their versions of what families had told them of the accidents. These parents were in awkward positions with regard to the burn unit, since they were now suspected of child abuse or neglect, it made visiting their children uncomfortable. Some of these parents saw their children only rarely, some not at all, and others, while visiting somewhat regularly, did not involve themselves in the daily recovery care of their children. They did not help with tubbings, dressing changes, and other play and recreation activities.

Observations did not indicate that staff attitudes or behaviors were directed toward discouraging these parents from the unit. In fast, the opposite seemd to be true. The nursing staff were pleased when these parents did visit their children and nurses were careful to explain all that was being done to and for their children. Likewise, nurses tended to get upset and discouraged when parents stayed away or visited infrequently.

As on the adult unit, the children's nurses were faced with the compliance problem: getting the children to endure the daily tubbings; persuading them to eat as much as they could; and, especially with the ambulatory children, seeing to it that the children behaved appropriately. Nursing philosophy on the children's unit was that the family role was crucial in this compliance process in that children were more likely to be swayed by parent's inducements than those of the staff. Additionally, nurses were sensitive to the problem of children's separation anxiety, thus, it was also the staff's philosophy that the rather constant and active presence of parents and family could reduce the fears and anxieties associated with the hospital experience and trauma of the burn injury.

The overt encouragement of family involvement in the many and varied aspects of burn recovery meant, however, that staff had to confront rather directly the parenting skills, interests, and degree of eagerness of the families. That is: how capable were these parents in assisting the staff with the recovery of their children and how eager and committed were they to the idea? Moreover, as we have seen, the problem was complicated further, as the staff recognized that many of these children came from broken homes; single, female-head-of-household, and in a significant number of cases the parents themselves were implicated in the burn injury of their child.

The result of these concerns was the tendency of staff to make a variety of evaluative judgments about the families of burn children. Staff went to considerable lengths to get a profile on the kinds of parents and families with whom they were dealing. Much of this took place during the child's first day of admission to the unit and the first few days subsequent to that. Nurses were especially concerned about the burn "story," how the accident happened, who was there, was there negligence, etc. In the first several days of a child's hospitalization the story was circulated repeatedly in nursing shift reports, team conferences and other occasions where nurses got together. No detail was considered too trivial and there was much concern that the story was "straight," that is to say, accurate and complete as possible.

Furthermore, nursing staff looked for many behavior and attitudinal clues as to the personal make-up of the family members themselves. Nurses were sensitive to behaviors that indicated the intelligence of families; the degree to which families were "with it," this is, aware of what was going on around them; and how much control they had over their children. Nurses also tried to perceive the amount of emotional bonding that existed between parents and children. Ideally, nurses had in mind a level of bonding in which parents were protective and aware of the child's needs for security and acceptance. Parents that appeared overprotective at the one extreme or indifferent to their children at the other, caused the nursing staff to regard them with wariness and concern, since staff would not expect problems in the involvement process.

Despite the amount of staff talk about these families and their competencies, skills and preparedness as parents or surrogates, nurses tended to be rather open and accepting of the families in terms of their daily interactions. While a number of the parents did not measure up to the staff's ideal, nurses for the most part accepted these parents as they were. If the families appeared interested in the welfare of their children and were willing to get involved in some level of the child's recovery care, and were able to exercise some degree of control over their child's behavior, then nurses openly embraced them into the social fabric of the burn unit.

A family-like atmosphere was created, nurses addressed all parents on a first name basis and introduced themselves likewise. Children's birthdays were celebrated with gusto and the nurses made several attempts to make the burn unit less threatening for the patients. Since many of the parents were very poor and often miles from their homes and extended families, the nurses and social worker saw to many of their basic food and shelter needs. Parents could draw from a special burn unit fund for food vouchers redeemable at the hospital cafeteria and nurses willingly permitted parents to sleep in the rooms with their children if other lodging could not be found.

Surgeons were much less interested in these families dynamics. A staff surgeon admitted to me he didn't "interface" much with the families of burn children because they rarely asked him intelligent questions. He preferred to leave the "interfacing" to the social worker, nurses and psychology consultants. The nursing staff, as a result, became rather close to several of these families as their children had repeated hospital stays on the burn unit for reconstructive surgeries, years after their original admission. Nurses were sent pictures of children on their birthdays and at times informed of a divorce or remarriage of one or more of the parents.

Encouraging a deeper level of parental involvement as a method for insuring compliance and reducing separation anxiety was not without its problems, however. The constant and active presence of families on the unit often upset routines and procedures. The over-involved and non-involved families both presented problems for the nurses and therapists. For example, during nursing report at shift change one of the evening shift nurses, Darlene, complained to her day shift colleagues who were coming on duty, "You know little Angela's (one and a half years old) parents just smother her! You have to apologize for going to Angela's room to give her medicine or something. If it was up to them they would do everything themselves. They even want to change all her diapers!"

In the above illustration we have one of the problems of parental over-involvement. The nurses didn't want parents to take over the care of their children completely! The "smothering" parent was an affront to the nursing staff's conception of their role and their own competence in caring for the children. The case below highlights yet another problem nurses faced when parent's attitudes and actions threatened nursing authority.

The parents of Wanda, an 8 year old girl, were members of a religious sect that rejected the use of medical science in the treatment of illness. Wanda was one of 6 children living in a home without electricity and running water. The family boiled water in large kettles for bathing and cooking and Wanda accidently pulled one of the kettles over on top of her. She sustained third degree scald burns to her chest, neck and arms, but her parents did not seek medical attention for her until 3 days after the accident. When Wanda was transferred to the burn unit she was critically ill. Her mother spent a good deal of time and with her in the hospital but her religious values and subsequent behaviors caused the staff much concern.

Darlene, one of the nurses was upset today at shift change, "You're not going to believe what Wanda's mom told her last night! She said that if Wanda prayed real hard she wouldn't need surgery in the monring! Can you believe that? Well . . . it really got Wanda upset and she was crying. Julie (one of the other night shift nurses had a talk with Wanda and told her that it was O.K. to pray, but the doctors and nurses were there to help too."

When parents were ambivalent about getting involved, this also disturbed work routines on the unit. The next case, taken from field notes, is rather lengthy, but demonstrates some of the problems parents and nurses faced in this ambivalency.

Susie was a one and a half year old child who suffered third degree scald burns to her legs, feet and toes when her mother left her and her brother alone for a short while in the bath tub. While her mother was in the bedroom getting their pajamas, the four year old turned on the hot water and jumped from the tub. Susie had a difficult hospital stay; as a result of her burns she was critically ill for a lengthy time due to metabolic disorders and electrolyte imbalances. Susie received critical care for several weeks and was immobilized and confined to bed. Georgia, her mother, stayed in her room constantly at first, but eventually became upset as Susie showed no signs of improvement and seemed so unresponsive to the world around her. Georgia began sitting outside Susie's room, making frequent trips to the hospital canteen, and gradually avoided going into Susie's room entirely. The nurses in addition to giving Susie intensive and continuous medical care soon found that she would scream anytime she was left alone even for a few minutes. They became frustrated with Georgia's refusal to spend time in Susie's room and they found themselves having to take turns being with her around the clock. Several of the nurses admitted to me, however, their feeling that Georgia needed a lot of "TLC" herself. Georgia, while refusing to go into her daugher's room also feared leaving the burn unit as she was in the process of getting a divorce from her husband and was concerned that, because of the circumstances surrounding Susie's scald injury, she might be accused of negligence and lose custody of her children. Both the sentimental order of the unit as well as the nursing routines were severely tested as Georgia remained on the unit for days, refusing to go further away than the canteen just down the hall, but also, resisting getting involved in Susie's care by staying out of her room! Thus a very awkward and difficult situation was created for the nurses and Georgia alike. Her continued presence on the ward, but her reluctance to get involved caused the nurses to not only see to Susie's continuous and serious medical needs, but also to give their constant physical presence to Susie in place of her mother.

This situation was unchanged for several days, and was only abated when Susie's condition gradually improved along with her disposition. As heart monitors, IV lines and catheters were removed and as Susie appeared more "normal," Georgia returned to the room and spent more time with her. Interestingly, a few months after Susie was allowed to go home, she and Georgia returned to the unit again for surgical reconstruction on Susie's feet. Several of the nurses remarked how much more relaxed Georgia seem to be with Susie and how much better she was getting along with the nurses. The unit social worker attributed this to the fact that Georgia's divorce was completed and had her life more together now.

Fathers and other male relatives were not as likely to involve themselves in the recovery care of children, but some fathers did spend time visiting their children and they often appeared bewildered and confused by the strangeness of the critical care setting.

Tommy was a two year old who was scalded on 20 per cent of his body when he pulled a crock pot on him while his mother was cooking. His mother was in the advanced stages of pregnancy when Tommy was brought to the burn unit, but she stayed with him most of the time. Tommy's father, Lee, was out of work and remained home to look for a job and care for the other two children at home. We would appear at unpredictable times, but the nurses were pleased when he showed considerable interest in Tommy's condition and chances for recovery.

Arlene was Tommy's nurse one evening and she reported to the other nurses at shift change, "Tommy's Dad showed up last night at 1:00 a.m. and want to pat Tommy. He ended up staying all night! I didn't mind it — but he woke Tommy up when he came in and we had just gotten him to sleep. Dad had a lot of questions and he kept asking me if it was O.K. to ask these questions about Tommy. I told him . . . 'Yes, these were good and appropriate questions.' However, I wish they hadn't been at 3:00 in the morning! But you know . . . even though Dad only finished the tenth grade, he has a good mind and doesn't seem that slow."

Nurses were most concerned that the mother or another female take the most active role in the recovery care of their children. In fact, nurses were somewhat surprised when fathers showed unusual interest in their children or when fathers had important questions to ask. Fathers were not discouraged from getting involved, it was more to the point that they were not expected to. When Lee showed up to spend the night with Tommy and had several insightful questions to ask it was so contrary to nurses expectations that Arlene included it in her report at shift change! Nurses would not have considered such behavior by Tommy's mother unusual at all — they would have expected it.

Some families got involved too quickly and completely in the care of their children and caused the nursing staff to assert itself as the legitmate authority in decision-making.

Two young girls, ages eight and twelve, from a Mennonite family were burned in an explosion during a camping trip. The girls were placed in the same room so they could be near each other. The mother and grandmother of the girls spent a good deal of their time with them, in fact, nurses were a little displeased to find that the grandmother and mother could hardly be persuaded to leave the room at all! Part of the protectiveness of the mother might have been due to her apprehensiveness about the "worldliness" of the hospital room with its television set, radio and other modern technology. While both the grandmother and mother were friendly and coopera- tive with the staff, they intended to be clearly in charge of the girls, seeing to it that they minded, ate their food, etc. At one point, the surgery resident took the mother aside and told her, "You don't have to push the girls so hard to eat their food. They are getting alot of IV fluids and that is plenty. Later we'll worry about their eating, O.K.?"

The Mennonite family presented no particular problems for the staff after the ground rules became established that the nurses and residents were in charge. Nurses were always careful to draw the dis- tinction between a family's becoming involved in the care of their child and their taking over in an authoritative sense. Burn unit staff welcomed the former and discouraged the latter.

In summary, the child of the family was really the child of the burn unit at least while the patient was in the emergent and acute phases. Though the nursing staff attempted to normalize the child's life as much as possible by permitting parents unlimited visiting privileges and encouraging their participation in much of the daily care of the child, nonetheless, the status of the child as a critically burned patient ultimately meant that the medical, nursing and therapy definitions of what was best for the child were ascendant. In the final analysis it was up to the parents and family to walk a rather narrow line between too little involvement with the child's recovery, which was interpreted as indifference; and over-involvement which tended to threaten the nurse's sense of authority and competence.

Conclusion

In this chapter we have seen some of the ordeals and stresses faced by burn victims and their families during the long arduous re- covery in the burn unit. The chapters to follow, shift our attention to the burn unit staff; the problems they face in helping burn patients recover and how they cope and come to terms. I begin my analysis of this process by examining the phenomenon of pain work, the many and varied ways that staff confront the pain experiences of their patients.

Chapter Four

PAIN WORK AMONG THE BURNED

PHIL Richards was the first patient that morning to go to the tank room for hydrotherapy and dressing change. It promised to be a busy morning for his nurse, Vicky, and Joan, the physical therapist, as the adult burn unit was at capacity and several patients would have to be brought to the tank for hydrotherapy before visiting hours at eleven o'clock.

In his late hirties, Phil was a muscular and powerfully built mechanic and part-time farmer, who had been burned on nearly 50 percent of his body when his tractor exploded. He lay now in the large hydrotherapy tank, submerged to the top of his shoulders in water heated to body temperature. His burns which covered much of his arms, chest, neck and hands were deeply reddened and raw looking; some areas of the upper arms were cracked and peeling. As Phill soaked quietly in the water, Vicky and Joan were busily breaking open packages of small pads what would be used to clean the burned areas on Phil's body. Both women worked quickly and silently, their faces were covered with masks and green hair nets fitted loosely over the tops of their heads. They wore surgical gloves on their hands and had tied yellow isolation gowns over their scrub suits. As the cleaning pads were tossed into the water, Joan and Vicky moved to opposite sides of the tank and knelt down to begin their work.

The portable radio, tuned to a rock station, was on fairly loud and the tank room itself was warm and humid. Phil looked uncomfortable and anxious despite the fact that the warm water was somewhat soothing on his burned skin. He turned his head to Vicky, "Please go easy this morning, I'm so sore." Vicky reassured him that they would go slow, and she asked him to lift his left arm out of the water so she could begin cleaning his burns. Joan began to dab with one of the pads at Phil's right shoulder at the same moment that Vicky started on his left arm, and within momemts Phil was squirming in the water with his legs flailing and thrashing. His face was soon contorted and misshapen as he held his breath. Joan quickly stopped and told him, "Phil, don't hold your breath like that, it's not good for your heart." Phil responded in a strained voice, "I can't help it. It just hurts so damn much!" Vicky reached out for his left hand which had been badly burned in the explosion, "Phil, you have to take some deep breaths. That's the only thing that will help in here. Take slow deep breaths and you'll start to relax." Phil responded, "It hurts too much to breathe, it's too much pain at once." Vicky, "Well you have to try, Phil."

Joan and Vicky continued their cleaning and after trying some deep breaths, Phil began to thrash more violently in the water. He was now moaning and soon the moans were louder than the music from the radio and the noise of the clanking water pipes. At other times, in the nearly twenty minutes Phil was in the tank, he would stop moaning and open his eyes and mouth wide as if he were going to scream, but no sounds followed. All at once he said loudly to Joan, "Please don't rub that spot on my elbow anymore! I'm just so sore there. Can't you work on some place else and go back to that? My whole arm there is the worse part!" Joan answered firmly, "O.K. Phil, I'll do your stomach now. But you know before we're through, I'll have to come back to your arm."

Neither Vicky nor Joan spoke much to Phil that morning, other than an occasional direction to raise or lower his arm. However, when the cleaning was finished, Joan leaned over the tank and said to Phil, "It's a good thing you're getting grafted (skin) tomorrow Phil, it will cover up some of those open spots. You won't be so sore after that." Phil nodded in silence, as if too weak to respond or even look pleased. He was glad to be finished with the cleaning and look forward to getting his fresh dressings put on and a chance to return to his room for a short rest before visiting hours.

Later that same morning I asked Joan why Phil's surgery would help reduce his pain. "Well Phil has a lot of open areas now and his burns are starting to heal. But that means the nerves are more exposed and when we clean those areas they really get sore. That's why he has so much pain now and I'm so glad they're taking him to surgery. You see as patients heal in, that's a sign of progress for us but it means a lot of pain for the patient."

That afternoon when visiting hours were concluded I went into Phil's room and found him laying quietly in bed. Except for his face and head he was wrapped in white gauze dressings and his arms were strapped in splints extending away from his body. He looked sleepy, but I asked him if he wanted to talk and he agreed. He looked up at me and said nearly in a whisper, "You know, it's something what some fellers have to suffer through." I pulled a chair up along one side of his bed and answered, "I guess you had a rough time in the tank this morning Phil." He nodded, "I didn't sleep good last night. For some reason they didn't give me a shot before I went to bed and I couldn't sleep. Whenever I can't sleep, it always seems to go worse back there (tank)." I asked him, "How do you feel now Phil?" "Oh not too bad. I just don't know what to think. I wonder if the other fellers show as much pain as I do. I told Joan this morning that my pain threshold is low. I know they tell you to relax, but how can you relax when it hurts so bad? Can you tell me?" I shook my head, "I don't know Phil. But it seems to me the others have as much pain as you do. I wouldn't worry about it." Phil looked at me, "Well I hope they give me something so I can sleep tonight. I've got surgery in the morning you know. Joan says that will help and I hope to God it does."

The daily pain-filled experiences of Phil Richardson, who was a patient on the burn unit for two months, were typical of most of the burn patients I observed. Recovery from a burn injury is above all a very painful ordeal. In this chapter I will analyze the place and meaning of pain in burn recovery, attempting to locate our understanding of pain within the more general problem of control; that is, the staff's need to control their work routines; and the patient's need to exercise some control over their pain experiences.

Patients on the burn units suffered intense physical pain, which was partially a result of their burn injury and partially due to the painful procedures involved in their recovery care. These latter procedures were especially numerous and included pain associated with: frequent blood tests, insertion of intravenous lines, dressing changes, the daily tubbings and laying immobile for hours in uncomfortable positions. Daily exercising of stiffened joints and tight burned skin was also a painful ordeal for patients, who dreaded their exercises almost as much as their morning sessions in the tank room. In addition, and as part of the dressing change routine, patients had to endure the pain of debridement which involved the removal of the dead burned skin, a process that activated the nerves along the edges of the living tissue. Moreover, as we saw in chapter three, partial thickness burns often left nerve endings intact and some patients experienced constant burning sensations.

Part of the responsibilities then of the nurses and therapists on the adult burn unit was in helping patients work through their pain. They did this in large measure by forcing patients to accept their pain experiences as given and essentially unalterable. In many ways, by words and actions, therapists and nurses communicated the following message to patients: "Yes, you are in pain, but there is nothing much that can be done about it. Only in pain will you heal and only in pain will you recover. On the burn unit it is O.K. to be in pain; we accept your pain because we accept you. But your pain cannot be an excuse; it won't prevent us from doing what we have to do." Put differently, burn unit staff tried to get patients to accept the inevitability of pain, but at the same time to reject the idea that pain could be limiting factor. In essence, this was what was meant by patients working through their pain: to recognize and accept the pain experience, but to come to terms with it by cooperating fully with staff in the recovery process.

As we shall see momentarily, no patients could use their pain as an excuse for avoiding exercises, dressing changes or the daily tubbings. Adult patients were expected to push themselves to their physical limits and to endure their pain with little complaining and only limited hope for relief. In the burn unit life was to go on, recovery work was to be accomplished and patients were pushed to rehabilitate themselves despite whatever pain and discomfort they might experience. So strong was this ideal of patients accepting their pain, that patients often verbally absolved the nurses of responsibility when their work caused patients to be in pain.

One morning during nursing report on the adult unit, Agnes, a nurse who had been working the evening shift, told her nursing colleagues about the behavior that evening of Lonnie, a teen-age patient, "It was really kind of funny last night, every time I did something painful to Lonnie, I would appologize because I knew it did hurt him. But he kept repeating, 'That's O.K. You're just doing your job aren't you?' Now that's kind of unusual for him. I wonder where he got that?" Sheri, a day shift nurse, smiled and said, "He got that from me because over the week-end, he started complaining whenever we tried to do something for him. So I told him we were just doing our job and we weren't trying to hurt him. He must have really taken that to heart!"

While burn unit patients were ideally expected to endure and accept their pain experiences, in reality, nurses and therapists endeavored to help patients come to terms with their pain. In order to ensure that nursing and therapy work could be carried out routinely, smoothly and with minimum disruptions and in ways that were somewhat emotionally satisfying, the pain experiences of patients had to be recognized and dealt with. While not all patients experienced the same levels of pain intensity and tolerance, and patients varied with respect to their fears of pain, it was up to the staff to structure and give meaning to the pain experiences of patients as if they were uniform and predictable. Thus, the nurses and therapists created a social context of pain work; norms, values and social routines that defined the meaning of pain on the burn unit and guided patients through the various pain-inducing aspects of their hospital recovery. All of this had to do with the ways in which nurses and therapists helped patients cope with their recovery in general, and in particular, come to terms with their pain experiences.

Helping patients to endure their pain, can be analyzed and understood within four broad coping strategies employed by therapists and nurses in structuring the pain experiences and responses of patients. I intend to introduce the strategies briefly here and to discuss them in detail in the pages to follow. I refer to the four coping strategies as: the pain contract; neutralizing the pain environment; giving patients control; and patient socialization. Briefly, the pain contract referred to a verbal and written understanding between patients and nurses for daily pain medication in which patients could choose the times and amounts of pain pills in a twenty-four hour period. Neutralizing the pain environment involved a variety of social and psychological techniques used by the burn unit staff to make the physical space or setting of the burn unit appear less threatening and fearful for burn patients. Giving patients control referred to a process whereby patients were given increased latitude and responsibility in controlling their own pain experiences and reponses. And finally, patients were taught, both directly and indirectly, how to deal with their pain in ways consistent with the social norms and values of the unit as a social setting. Having introduced these strategies, I would now like to focus attention on each one in more detail. We will start with an analysis of the pain contract.

The Pain Contract

Burn units in the United States are known to vary with respect to the kind and amounts of pain medication that are prescribed for burn patients. One of the most powerful and effective pain relief drugs, morphine, is commonly used on most hospital burn units, but, again, the strength and frequency of dosages is subject to considerable variability.

At the time of study, the adult burn unit being investigated here, used morphine rather sparingly and did not employ morphine injections routinely during dressing changings and daily tubbings. With minor variations, the same policy was in effect on the children's unit. Typically, the surgery residents wrote standing pain medication orders, that included morphine injections during the patients' first few days on the burn unit. Assuming that the patient made normal progress toward recovery, including being fluid resuscitated, regaining consciousness, etc., patients were taken off morphine near the end of their first week of admission. Subsequent to that, patients received daily oral pain medications that were far less powerful and effective than morphine.

Part of the reasoning behind this philosophy had to do with the physical effects of morphine which tends to depress a patient's respirations, which was a concern in treating patients suffering from inhalation injuries. Equally important for our purposes here were the experiences of burn unit staff who held that dosages of morphine sufficient to totally alleviate a patient's pain, would also render them virtually unconscious or at the least, incapable of actively participating in the recovery program. In other words, if patients were going to do for themselves, engage in their daily exercises, take in several thousand calories per day in food, and normalize their lives as much as possible while in the burn unit, they had to be somewhat physically and mentally alert. Large amounts of morphine were considered to be counter productive to patients' vigorous participation in the life of the setting because of the physiological effects of such a powerful drug. Moreover, many nurses on the adult burn unit thought morphine to be an addictive drug, and were reluctant to ask surgeons for morphine orders due to their fears of patient addiction. In the case of dying patients, none of the above reasons were in effect, and morphine was used routinely to keep such patients comfortable and pain free.

Thus, patients on the adult burn unit could count on morphine for pain relief only during the emergent or critical care phase. Subsequent to that, patients received oral pain medications of varying degrees of strength, none of which, in the opinions of burn unit staff and patients alike, were strong enough to totally alleviate pain. As one nurse expressed it, "The kind of pain medications we've been giving just sort of take the edge off. It's about what you and I would take for a tooth-ache. They sure don't do much for burn pain." In addition to pain medications, surgeons occasionlly wrote orders for tranquilizers, usually at the request of nurses, for those patients whose tensions and anxieties seemed to worsen their pain. Normally, these orders were only temporary, lasting for only a few days at a time, as a stop-gap measure to help certain patients get accustomed to the daily tubbings and other painful procedures.

Most adult patients were put on a contract for their daily oral pain medications. The contract was written into the nursing care plan and became part of the patient's official record. Nurses carefully explained the details of the contract to patients and the typical contract called for a patient to receive twelve to sixteen pain pills a day and no more. The contractual agreement allowed patients to choose the times of day when they would receive their pills, two at a time.

Nurses made very explicit to patients the terms of the contract; that sixteen pills were the absolute daily limit, and that once a patient requested two pills, for example, at nine in the morning, she/he could not ask for additional pills an hour later. Though patients were free to choose the times they wanted their pain medication, there had to be sufficient time between medication periods to ensure that patients would not overdose and that there would be enough pills to get them through the evening hours.

Without the nurses having to tell them, most patients learned very quickly when their most painful daily periods were and these periods normally centered around their two daily dressing changes, their exercise sessions with the therapists, and during the evening as patients attempted to rest and sleep. Thus most patients learned to space their pain medications throughout the day and evening and most would request two pain pills before and after their morning session in the hydrotherapy tank and dressing change; two pills before and after their afternoon exercises with the occupational therapist, and similarly, pills accompanying evening dressing changes and before sleep. While most patients learned this routine on their own, sometimes nurses suggested this structure to them in negotiating the contracts during their first week on the unit.

The use of the pain contract was thought to be a means of giving burn patients some control over their pain destiny. Most nurses favored the contract because it allowed patients the freedom to determine some aspects of their pain experiences and likewise gave patients a sense of independence. Both parties, nurses and patients alike, were bound by the terms of the contract. Patients did not have to beg for favors in getting pain medications, since by terms of the contract, this was something that was their due and nurses were obligated to honor their request. From the viewpoint of the nurses, patients could no longer make unreasonable demands for pain pills, as the paients knew the rules as well as the staff. In this sense, when a nurse decided not to honor a patient's request, it was not so much the nurse saying "No" to a patient, but, rather one partner in an argreement reminding the other of the contractual terms.

Eric White was a twenty-one year old patient with full thickness burns to his right arm and shoulder. Normally, he tried not to show much pain, especially when he was in the company of the four other young male patients who were in the burn unit during his tenure. Eric was considered handsome by the nurses and he frequently tried to use his appealing looks to gain favors from the nurses. On this morning, toward noon, Eric had been complaining of burning sensations up and down his right arm. From his chair in the television lounge, he spotted his nurse June as she was hurrying down the hall, "June, my arm is really sore this morning. Can't I have two more of my pills?" June stopped and said in a stern voice, "Eric you know better than to ask. We've been over this before. You've had your quota for this morning and that's that." She then turned and proceeded down the hall. Later in the television lounge Eric complained to William, another young male patient. "God, I don't like June at all. She won't give an inch, and I don't know why I keep getting stuck with her as my nurse."

Such examples as the above were not infrequent; the pain contract did not always negate the fact that patients who were in constant pain often wanted to toss the contract aside temporarily and try to cajole the staff into extra medication. While patients understood the terms of the contract, there were occasions when their pain seemed worse than usual and thus they resorted to asking the staff to make exceptions.

While nurses rarely gave in to such requests, the surgery residents, who made daily round to briefly examine patients, often went along with what patients might ask for. Residents were sometimes unaware that a patient was at quota, or they were so busy making rounds that it was easier to give patients extra pain medications than it was to argue with them or go into lengthy explanations of the rules. Some patients came to learn which of the residents were most agreeable on this matter and would routinely ask the resident for an extra allotment in defiance of their nurses.

As might be expected, staff nurses resented the residents ordering additional pain medication for patients, but there was little they could do about it other than to remind the resident about the importance of the contract. Occasionally this worked and the resident would change her/his mind and so inform the patient. However, since only the nurse and the patient were bound by the contract, surgery residents tended to do what was most expedient and convenient at the moment a patient request was made.

In summary, the pain contract was a method whereby the nursing staff gave patients some control over their pain by providing a structure of pain medication timetables that allowed each patient the latitude to decide when some measure of relief was most important and crucial. Patients were afforded the ability to tailor their medication according to their individual needs and the unique personal daily rhythms of their own pain. From the standpoint of the nursing staff, the contract removed some of the arbitrariness from the nursing role and permitted nurses to dispense pain medications in an even-handed and impersonal way. It tended to eliminate potential nurse/patient conflicts that could have arisen if patients felt that nurses were playing favorites or showing partiality in allocating pain medication. As we will see in the next chapter, the pain contract also restricted the use of pain pills to control patient behavior on the unit.

Neutralizing the Pain Environment

The second coping strategy employed by burn unit staff in structuring the pain experiences and responses of patients, I refer to as neutralizing the pain environment. As can be seen in the previous section, nurses and therapists had somewhat limited medication resources to help patients control their pain. Morphine use was restricted, and the number of other oral pain medications available were never strong enough to completely eliminate the pain experienced by most patients. In light of this, staff created ways to make the burn unit setting itself appear less like a painful environment. Part of this had to do with subtle but important modifications in the physical environment; other methods were associated with staff demeanor, attitudes and styles of action and relations with patients. While the burn units themselves were rather somber hospital wards where a good deal of human suffering and pain took place, the burn staff attempted to counter the primary social definition of the burn unit as a place of serious and critical medical work with a secondary definition of the environment as a pleasant, optimistic, almost cheerful and normal place to be. By manipulating the physical setting and employing counter social themes and definitions the staff worked to get patients to think less about their pain and suffering and to embrace the upbeat and optimistic ideals of the setting. I would like to look more closely now at how the staff sought to accomplish this.

While the physical and ecological settings of the two burn units were essentially fixed, there were a variety of small but significant ways that staff employed to change the stark and austere nature of the wards. On the adult unit the tub room with the massive hydrotherapy tank and dressing carts was a setting of great pain and suffering for patients who were brought their daily for hydrotherapy and dressing changes. This room though fairly large, was usually very warm and humid and patients often could be heard loudly moaning, groaning and even screaming throughout their hour-long session there. Many patients came to fear the time spent in that room and the nurses and therapists tried to distract the patients' sense of suffering by playing the radio in the room the entire morning. The music was turned up loud, because it had to cover up the sounds of water splashing in the tank and the banging of the ancient water pipes. Nurses encouraged patients to choose their favorite radio stations, or type of music before the hydrotherapy was to begin. During the musical numbers there were jokes and kidding remarks between staff and patients about whether anyone felt like dancing and who on the burn unit was the best dancer or singer.

Similarly, on the large door leading into the tank room was a good-sized poster drawn up by the nurses that read, "You Are Now Entering Tub City U.S.A." And on the inside of the door leading out of the tank room, where patients passed though after their dressing change there was a corresponding sign reading, "You Are Now Leaving Tub City, U.S.A. We Hope Your Stay Was a Pleasant One." Most patients grimly acknowledged the ironic humor of that sign, in that for at least another day, their journey to the tub room was now over.

Burn unit staff also sought to inspire patients to be optimistic and courageous in the painful recovery process and they adorned the walls and doors of the burn unit with inspirational posters. These posters were composed of large colorful photos of landscapes and pastoral scenes, and beneath each photo or painting were inspiring messages such as the following: "Happiness is found along the way, not at the end of the road."

Additionally, patients on the adult unit were encouraged to decorate their rooms with any pictures, cards, photographs or ornaments that would give the space a more home-like or human atmosphere. For those patients on the unit for several months the walls of their rooms became collage of cards, posters and even pin-up displays. IV poles were used to hang balloons and colorful mobiles, although this device was more common on the children's unit.

The staff in the burn unit designated for children went to considerable lengths to transform hospital space into essentially child's space. As described earlier in Chapter Two, the children's unit was continually decorated with large mobiles, balloons, and child-oriented pictures. Children were permitted to play with all of the toys and games from the toy shelves and much of the play took place on the floor of the unit so that staff and visitors had to walk rather carefully when play was in session. Mobiles were also hung over the beds of children, especially those still confined to bed in the emergent phase. Children were able to bring stuffed animals and dolls to bed with them and nurses and visitors would read stories to those children in bed.

Parents and close relatives could visit on a twenty-four hour basis and family-centered activities and play were encouraged by the nurses. The tub rooms where children underwent their painful dressing changes, likewise were equipped with toys, and children could play with the rubber and plastic animals while soaking in the tub. The children's unit looked as much like a nursery school and playground as it did a hospital ward.

Along one hall of the children's unit, there was a large bulletin board with color pictures of the children; those presently hospitalized along with pictures of those who had gone home some months before. Beneath each picture were written humorous and sentimental captions that personalized each child's picture. Nurses were quick and eager to take the children's photos and while birthdays and special holidays provided almost certain picture-taking, nearly every child made the picture board at some time during his/her stay.

Older children were encouraged to watch television in their rooms as a diversion and the nurses occasionally watched programs with them. In fact, nurses on the children's ward often played with the youngsters as a way of developing trust and engaging children to interact with them in non-painful contexts. One afternoon when there were few visitors and medical staff on the unit two of the nurses and I played a version of indoor soccer with Felix, a twelve-year old boy who had massive scald burns to his thighs and buttocks. This activity was designed not only to divert his attention from his pain, but, also, to overcome his reluctance to exercise his legs which was important at that stage of his recovery.

Examination of nursing care plans on the children's unit revealed the nurses recognized the importance of diversionary activities for children. On one care plan for two sisters, eight and ten years old, their nurse, Jackie, had recommended "doing fun things" with the children in addition to medication as a way of helping the young girls cope with their pain. The sisters were also allowed to share the same room to lessen separation anxiety and promote a home-like atmosphere for them.

Aside from modifications of the physical environment of the burn-care setting, staff helped patients deal with pain through the use of teasing and humor. Though the work performed on patients was complex, complicated and usually painful, such actions were approached and undertaken in a light-hearted, open and friendly way. Both patients and staff knew that dressing changes, debridement, and hydrotherpay exercises would be very painful and uncomfortable, but staff prodded patients to focus their attention on more pleasant and less stressful themes and subjects. While a patient's pain was acknowledged in the course of a dressing change, it was not dwelled upon, and staff attempted to draw patients out in humor and teasing. The following cases are taken from fieldnotes on the adult unit.

After an especially painful session in the hydrotherapy tank, Phil Richardson was laying on the dressing cart, while Anne, the physical therapist, began picking at the dead skin along the burned surfaces of his arms and shoulder. Phil winced and groaned out load as Anne slowly and carefully peeled away layers of skin. At one point Phil said to Anne, "You know I'm feeling something." Anne asked him, "What do you feel like Phil?" "I almost feel like smacking you," Phil replied. Anne grinned at him, "Oh don't do that to me." Phil managed a smile, "I'm just kidding, you know that." Anne wiggled a finger at him, "Well you better be Phil. Because we'll just smack you right back. We're tough around here."

On another occasion in the tank room, Ned Rice, a foundry worker severely burned in an explosion was nearly finished with his dressing change. Ned had remained pretty quiet this hour in the tank room, but after a while he started to keep time to the music on the radio and Vickie, his nurse, asked me to turn the volume up. Vickie was helping Ned get into a fresh pair of scrub pants and as she began to pull the draw string, she realized the pants were several sizes too large. Vickie laughed, "Ned there's room for you and me both inside these pants!" Ned grinned, "Well, I guess we could really dance together then, couldn't we?"

Nurses also used teasing themes for certain patients as a way of getting through a painful procedure. Such themes were employed for an entire morning or day and were an attempt to draw patients out of their silence or fears about impending activities. George Dunbar was sixty years old and critically burned in a home accident and was hospitalized for nearly three months with 50 per cent full and partial thickness burns. On this particular morning he was to go to the tank room after being confined to bed for several days with a serious infection. Gwenn, his nurse, was slowly helping him onto the cart from his bed when she noticed that his buttocks was warm and indented with marks from the bed sheets after having been in bed all night, Gwenn laughed out loud, "George, you've got Hot Cross Buns. You know that?" Gwenn kidded George about his Hot Cross Buns during the entire time in the tank room and several other nurses picked up on that theme in their interactions with George during the day.

On another occasion, when the movie "E.T." was popular, one of the patients, Mark, had mentioned that he had seen the movie several times. Mark also was noted for his sweet tooth and fondness for candy. While Mark was in the tank room one morning for hydrotherapy, two of the nurses found a package of chocolates and used them to spell out a large E.T. on Mark's freshly made bed. This was his greeting upon returning to his room later in the morning.

As I mentioned in a previous chapter, much of the work that nurses and therapists did for patients was pain inducing. One of the ways that staff came to terms with this aspect of their role was to joke and tease with each other and with patients about their "sadistic" tendencies. Sadism was jokingly referred to as the reason why staff liked to work in a burn unit in the first place.

Sarah, an occupational therapist was putting Gordon Miley through a series of range-of-motion exercises, getting Gordon to stretch his arms and shoulders which had been burned in a gasoline explosion. Gordon was a huskily built mechanic and accustomed to using his arms, but since his injury he could barely raise them above his head. Sarah was having Gordon place a pole in a rack several feet over his head. After trying for several minutes, Gordon's face was sweating, his mouth drawn tight in pain and his entire body was trembling. Gordon looked at Sarah and said, "This is making sweat break out on me." Sarah answered him smiling, "See Gordon, when you asked me why I went into this work; I like to hurt people." Gordon came back, "I thought you were a sadist." Sarah laughed, "Gee, I hope you know I'm only kidding."

George Dunbar was soaking in the hydrotherpay tank, while Vera, his nurse, was cleaning his burned skin. George turned to her, "Let me ask you Vera. Which do you like best, taking off my dressings or putting them on?" Vera replied, "Why George, you must think we're a bunch of sadists around here." George smiled weakly, "Well I'm not sure. I'm merely asking."

Gary, a twenty-two year old construction worker with 40 percent partial thickness burns to his arms and chest was resting on the dressing cart in the tank room as Joan, the physical therapist, and his nurse June, were putting on fresh gauze dressings over his wounds. June was looking closely at Gary's right arm, and asked Joan, "What is this dark crusted area here under his elbow?" Joan peered over the table at the spot and said, "Oh that's where we took his skin biopsy yesterday." Gary spoke up, "Yeah and they took half my body with it!" Joan laughed, "Now Gary, are you complaining about my surgery?"

The above examples also illustrate the light-hearted banter between staff and patients that characterized much of the interactions in the tank room. There were, of course, many serious moments and sometimes the work was done with little interpersonal exchange, but usually the staff liked to engage patients in conversation laced with good humor and ribbing. When patients insisted on being silent and withdrawn, the nurses and therapists chatted among themselves while they assisted each other in wound debridement and dressing changes. The morning sessions in the tank room were an occasion for staff to catch up on news and gossip and to discuss week-end activities and plans.

Because the tank room represented for patients such a stressful and painful environment and many patients were anxious about their session there each morning, nurses and therapists attempted to deemphasize the serious and foreboding nature of the room by their use of teasing and humor and employing a demeanor of competency and calmness. Moreover, staff tried to mask their own anxieties about inflicting pain, by relating to patients in a casual and calm, yet competent manner. A "business as usual" stance was taken by staff; they proceeded slowly and with care and tried not to react emotionally or get upset when patients began to cry, scream or beg to be left alone. By creating an aura of "all in a day's work," pain work was treated as normal and routine. As staff conveyed to patients the impression that there was nothing out of the ordinary in what they were doing, staff were able to deal with their own stresses and tensions. In turn, patient anxieties were lessened as they came to accept the prevailing definition of the situation and learned to live with their pain. The various medications helped patients somewhat, but their pain was also mitigated to a degree as they opened up to the joking and teasing and began to realize along with the staff, that by seeing things as normal, they weren't quite so bad after all.

Giving Patients Control

Turning now to the third coping stratgegy, I would like to explore how staff got patients to deal with their pain by enabling them to gain some measure of control over the pain experience. One of the sources of patients anxieties was the loss of control they felt during the period of hospitalization. This forced dependency is common, no doubt, among nearly all hospitalized adults, whose normal adult roles are temporarily suspended as they assume the patient role. With burn patients the problem was especially acute because their forced dependency and sense of helplessness heightened their anxieties which in turn increased their pain fears and even sensations. Nursing and therapy staff realized the relation between loss of control and heightened pain anxieties and tried to create ways in which patients could exercise some control, however limited, over their pain experiences. My observations revealed two general areas of patient control: the pain contract itself, and various attempts by patients to manipulate the painful aspects of their daily physical care.

We have already discussed the nature of the pain contract, but I want to re-emphasize here how patients' use of the contract allowed them to manipulate their pain. One important way this was accomplished was through the patients' ability to time their medications around the daily painful procedures to which they were subject. Each patient discovered which procedures, events and times of day brought the greatest pain, and the contract allowed them to receive and the nursing staff to allocate medication accordingly. As might be expected, once patients were accustomed to timing their pain medications, they were reluctant to accept any interruptions in their schedule.

Vince Rodman, a fifty-year old patient, was sitting in the television lounge smoking a cigarette nervously awaiting his turn in the tank room that morning. Joan, the physical therapist, walked out of the tank room looking for Vince and she spotted him in the lounge, "Vince, we're waiting for you now." Vince looked concerned, "Well, I just had the pills a few minutes ago and I'm waiting for them to take effect. I'd just as soon not be in pain." Joan asked him, "When did you take them?" "Five minutes ago, " Vince answered. Joan was firm with him, "Well, we have a lot of people to do in the tank this morning Vince, and you're first. We would like to finish before lunch." Vince was able to relax a few more minutes before Glenda, his nurse for that day, peeked into the lounge and said, "We're waiting for you." Vince slowly stood up, let out a deep sigh, and said to me, "I guess with all this peer pressure, I better get down there."

Val was a forty-five year old farmer who had been to surgery for skin grafting a week earlier. This was the morning that the nurses were going to remove the staples from his arms that held the grafts in place. Val and I were chatting in the television lounge when he said to me with a worried look on his face. "Sheri (his nurse) said that I can have my pain pills this morning before I get my staples out. I told her that was when I wanted them today. God, I hope she doesn't forget them, or give them to me before they can take effect!"

Nurses and therapists also allowed patients to gain control over the procedures or processes of their daily care that they considered most painful. Most of these routines or actions were not major activities, but patients considered them significant and important signs of independence. Such activities took the form of small bargaining agreements or negotiations in which patients traded greater cooperation with staff for limited opportunities to exercise control. The painful aspects of physical care in the tank room provided frequent opportunities for these bargaining agreements.

Ned Rice had just been lowered into the hydrotherapy tank and was submerged to his shoulders in warm water. He had sustained burns on 40 percent on his upper body. When he saw Vickie, his nurse, reach for the cleaning pad, as she knelt at the side of the tank, he said to her, "You're going to to let me soak here for awhile aren't you? It seems to go better that way." Vickie nodded and replied, "O.K. Ned, you can have a few minutes, but then we've got to get started."

Other patients insisted on some soaking time in the tank and would quickly remind the staff when there were promises or agreements to that effect. George Dunbar, who was often very straightforward with the burn unit staff, lay in the hydrotherapy tank for only a few seconds when Myra, the physical therapist, reached for his hand to start his exercises. George got emphatic with her, "Now Myra, you promised me this morning that I could soak in here for a few minutes, and I want every second of it!" Myra laughed, "O.K. George, you're right, I did promise. But you only get twenty minutes in the tank so you can't soak for very long."

Gene Morris was twenty years old and had sustained acute burns to his arms and shoulder in a grease fire. One day after he had been lowered into the tank, Lucille, the therapist activated a device in the tank that caused the water to bubble. Many patients found these bubbles very painful and Gene was soon crying and begged Lucille to stop the bubbles. She didn't at first, but as Gene's cries turned to sobs and shrieks of pain she disconnected the bubble device. Gene's crying subsided and he even managed to smile at her. Lucille leaned over to him, "Quit your smiling Gene, you're getting away with murder, you know that? You're really going to work now. Get those arms in the air." Gene did as he was told and went through his exercises with determination, but didn't complain or cry during the rest of his time in the tank.

Yet another way staff gave patients some control over their pain was to allow patients to do some of the painful procedures themselves. By permitting patients to perform their own work, patients could proceed at an individual pace and since they knew which parts of their bodies were sorest, patients applied pressure or gentleness accordingly. Thus patients while in the hydrotherapy tank often were handed cleaning pads and directed to clean their burn wounds themselves. This action occurred most often when patients had been on the unit for a week or more and were familiar with proper cleaning techniques. Those patients in the latter stages of the recovery process, who no longer required the hydrotherapy tank, but needed daily showers, were allowed to shower themselves and remove their own dressings. Patients looked forward to this privilege as they could adjust water pressures according to their level of comfort and remove the dressings at their own pace.

With respect to the latter, removal of dressings was often one of the most painful procedures burn patients had to endure. The gauze dressings wrapped over the antimicrobial creams that protected the burn wounds, dried out in six to ten hours and when these dressings were peeled off, they pulled loose the dead skin and opened up raw, tender, new skin underneath. On occasions, patients were given the chance to remove these dressings themselves, so that nurses were free from such a pain-inducing activity.

One afternoon I watched as Audry, a nurse, helped Sam Edwards remove his dressings and at one point, she said to him, "Sam, why don't you just take them off yourself? You know what to do. Then call me when you're ready for your shower." Later in the hall I asked her why she did that. Audry explained, "I let him go on his own, because it hurts. Sometimes it's better to let them hurt themselves. Sam gets the job done quickly, and doesn't take too much time. I poured a solution over the dressings so they will come off easier. Normally we don't do that because we want to debride as the dressings come off, but Sam is pretty well debrided now."

Giving patients some control over pain work served two functions in dealing with pain on the burn unit. One, this strategy lessened the nurses' and therapists' involvement in pain-inducement. As patients were directed to do some of their own work, they themselves became pain inflicters and that began to reduce some of the resentment that patients built up against the staff. More importantly, by giving patients more control in structuring their pain experiences, patients were drawn into the social fabric of the burn unit. This had the effect of abating patients' fears and anxieties about pain as they gained some small measure of independence by participating in their own pain work and physical care.

Patient Socialization

The final coping device used by burn unit staff in helping patients come to terms with pain had to do with a process of socialization in which patients learned appropriate pain responses and behaviors. This learning process was considered important by the staff for two reasons. One, as we have already discussed, patients' pain sensations often were heightened and intensified by fears and anxieties, which were due in part, to patients' lack of understanding about the importance and meaning of different pain sensations. Therefore staff recognized the importance of helping patients understand the various kinds of pain they were experiencing and the relationship between pain and the healing process itself. Two, since patient pain responses and behaviors could at times interfere with the smooth and routine nature of staff work, patients had to learn to express and come to terms with pain in ways that did not upset the orderly flow of routines on the burn unit. In other words, while it was acceptable for patients to express their pain, they had to learn to do it in ways that didn't bother other patients or disrupt the daily work of the burn unit staff. Thus patients learned two things on the burn unit with respect to pain: the meaning of their pain sensations, and behaviors and responses appropriate to the setting. I would like to look closely now at this socialization process.

When patients were first admitted to the burn unit, the staff were quite solicitous toward them about their pain. During the first few days, nurses and therapists frequently asked patients if they were in pain, and would also apologize to them if they caused a patient to wince or cry out. Nurses especially went to some lengths to explain the pain contracts for patients and reminded patients to ask for medication if they were getting uncomfortable. In these communications there was an early acknowledgement of pain by the staff, and patients soon realized that their pain was normal, expected and not temporary. Also patients learned that the staff did not expect them to endure their pain without some help in the form of pain medication. However, they also learned that their pain would not exempt them from all the activities they would have to engage in to bring about their recovery.

Interestingly some of the children on the children's unit often felt they were being punished for their burn accidents, especially if they were burned as a result of their own carelessness or mischief. Nurses on the children's unit had to carefully and continually remind such children that their painful tubbings and dressing changes were not forms of punishment for hurting themselves, but necessary procedures to help them get well. Learning for these children meant accepting the idea that their pain was not their own fault.

On the adult unit nurses took care to provide validation for a patient's pain, particularly when it was the nurse who was doing something painful to the patient. According to Audry, a nurse on the adult burn unit, "I feel it's important that we let patients know that we recognize their pain. In effect we tell patients, 'I know I'm hurting you and I know this is painful. But it is also necessary.' It's important too that patients learn that the nurse doesn't want to inflict pain. It's just something that can't be avoided. I tell my patients, 'I don't intentionally inflict pain on you. What I do has a purpose, but that purpose is not to give you pain!'"

In addition to the validation process, therapists and nurses saw to it that patients learned the various meanings of pain in so far as they were defined in that burned care setting. Here patients learned in a variety of ways and contexts the reasons for their pain and how different procedures and recovery stages would lessen or increase their pain.

Staff used the occasions of skin-grafting surgery to provide a benchmark of expectations for patients about their future pain. Surgeons and nurses encouraged patients to agree to skin-graft procedures for two different reasons, according to Glenda, one of the most experienced nurses on the burn unit. "Surgeons tell patients that a skin graft will shorten the amount of time they have to spend in the hospital. And that is usually true. But nurses tell patients that grafting will cover up their open areas and they won't have as much pain." Thus nurses encouraged patients to look forward to surgery because it represented a way of lessening their pain. Depsite this not all patients agreed to surgery and some patients' fear of surgery outweighed their concerns for the amount of pain they were experiencing.

Vickie, one of the day-shift nurses, walked into Gary's room to tell him how far behind he was that day on his calories. In his mid-twenties Gary was four weeks post-burn and his burned skin which covered parts of his chest and arms, was healing very slowly. Vickie was firm with him, "Gary you had only 100 calories for breakfast. This just isn't enough. You're going to have a chocolate malt now before lunch. You're not getting enough calories to help your skin heal!" Gary sat in his chair, with his head down. He appeared nervous and was shaking. "Well, I don't want any more surgery; I'll try to eat." Vickie moved closer to where Gary was sitting and leaned down toward his face. She said distinctly, "Gary, listen to me. Do you want all this pain? And keep asking for more pain pills. And a week from now they (surgeons) will look at you again and say you still need to be grafted. You're just putting it off!"

As we saw earlier, when burned skin begins to heal, pain sensations for patients increase as nerve endings push close to the surface with newly regenerating skin buds. While patients expected initially that as they improved physically, they should feel better, in reality, the opposite was true. As patients improved their pain intensified almost dramatically. Nurses helped patients prepare for this, as they informed them about the relationship between pain and healing.

It was a warm, muggy and noisy morning in the tank room and Ned Rice who was three weeks post-burn was squirming and thrashing in the hydrotherpay tank trying to avoid the touch of his nurse Vera who as cleaning his burn wounds. Ned was groaning loudly, but paused for a moment and in a tired and hoarse voice told Vera he just wanted to lay there. "Please don't scrub me now; I just want to sit for awhile." Vera answered, "Well, O.K. Ned, but I'll shave you while you're soaking. Ned squeaked, "No, don't shave me. I just couldn't stand it today." Vera insisted, "I'm afraid I have to Ned." Ned responded in a weak voice, "I don't know what's wrong. I'm just so sore today. I can't stand to be touched!" Vera looked at him over her mask and said quietly, "You're healing so good Ned and that makes you sore. The more you heal the more sore you're going to get."

During Monday Grand Rounds the entire burn unit staff had assembled in Phil Richardson's room and the surgeons were finishing examining his burn wounds which covered his chest, arms and hands. As they were filing past Phil's bed on their way out, Phil said to them barely above a whisper, "You know doctor, my pain is pretty bad; it seems to be worse." No one responded, but as Maureen, one of the nurses, walked by the foot of his bed she paused and said to Phil, "You're starting to close in now Phil, so you will be uncomfortable for awhile. But, you'll be O.K."

At other times patients were reminded that their present pain was necessary to avoid future complications and pain, and necessary to promote a quicker recovery. Such was the case with Ollie, a sixty-five year old patient, who suffered severe burns to his arms, chest and back in a house fire. Ollie had been hospitalized for over four months at the time of this study and was required to wear splints on his arms to keep his joints from contracting and losing his mobility. One day Sandi and Dale, the occupational therapists, had constructed a new splint for Ollie and in the process of adjusting it to him properly, caused Ollie a good deal of pain. During the fitting Ollie had screamed, sobbed, and turned red in the face as he nearly choked. As Sandi walked down the hall to get him a glass of juice, Dale tried to soothe Ollie's feelings. "Ollie, I know it hurts getting this splint fitted, but it's the only way to prevent more surgery if you get contractures. Sure it hurts now, but it will save you a lot of pain later."

Gordon Miley, a forty-year-old mechanic, was sitting in the television lounge with several of the nurses as he was telling them of his experiences the previous evening. "I had such severe pain in the shower last night that it brought me to my knees. You know that's the first time in my life when I had pain I couldn't stand." Glenda smiled at him and replied, "That happens to a lot of our patients. When you are first burned your body is so shocked you don't feel the pain. Later though you feel it more intensely."

Patients learned not only the meaning of pain and its relation to stages of recovery and healing, they also were socialized by staff to express their pain at appropriate times and placed. Nurses and therapists had definite ideas about when they expected patients to have the most pain and under what circumstances they would permit patients to express their pain openly and freely. Thus there were various norms in the burn unit about appropriate pain responses and expressions and patients had to learn these norms and conform to them if they were to win the approval of the staff. Burn unit nurses wanted work and activities to go smoothly and with a minimum of disruption and upset, and patients were socialized to express their pain in ways consistent with these values.

In the tank room, nurses and therapists expected patients to be in considerable pain and since the room was somewhat noisy and separated by two sets of doors from the rest of the burn unit, patients were permitted to scream and vocalize their pain sensations at will.

Bobby Williams was in his fourth week of hospitalization with 90 per cent body surface burns. He was twenty-three years old and injured in an explosion. Bobby had been taken to the tank room where Joan and Vera were unwrapping his dressings to get him ready for hydrotherapy. His legs were badly burned and as his dressings were peeled from his thighs, large amounts of dead skin were pulled off. Vera and Joan took several minutes to do this and Bobby's screams filled the room. He screamed at several levels of intensity, sometimes shrieking and moments later he would sob loudly and deeply. Throughout his screaming he would cry out periodically, "I know this has to done!" Joan and Vera worked silently and methodically on Bobby's legs without looking directly at him. Joan suggested several times that he take deep breaths. Finally, after several minutes Vera said, "We're almost finished Bobby, just hang on and you'll soon be in the water. You'll like that won't you? Art's got the water nice and warm for you."

In the above example, while Bobby screamed uncontrollably, Joan and Vera made no attempt to quiet him. This was partly because they knew that removing his dressings was excruciatingly painful and since he was burned 90 percent that was a terrific amount of pain for anyone to endure. Also, as they were in the tank room, it was permissible for Bobby to openly express his pain. Aside from this Bobby was considered a fairly cooperative patient throughout his tenure on the burn unit and was normally stoic in his response to pain. In fact he accepted the norms of the burn unit almost totally and even in his shrieking he reminded the nurses that he understood what they were doing, "I know this has to be done!"

Nurses were less likely to allow patients to scream and yell in their own rooms during dressings changes or while other nursing or therapy work was being performed. Such behaviors were thought to be upsetting to other patients and visitors on the unit and made the work of nurses and therapists more difficult. Even though the staff would close the door to the room when pain work was being done, patients were still expected to contain their vocal expressions.

During lunch in the nurses lounge, Vickie and Glenda were discussing Marcia, a woman patient in her fifties with severe burns to her face, neck and arms. She had been hospitalized for over a month and had undergone several skin-graft operations. Glenda remarked, "Marcia was doing a lot of complaining today in her room while we were trying to change her dresssings. I know her donors were sore when we took the dressings off them, but once she started yelling she wouldn't stop. She kept yelling, 'Hurry up and get me closed!' and I just said to her, 'Not until you stop hollering! We're not going to put up with it.' "

On other occasions patients learned indirectly that their complaints of pain were becoming inappropriate, and while the staff would help them up to a point, beyond that patients had to learn self control. The next two cases illustrate this idea.

In the tank room, June was debriding the burn wounds of Bob Quinn, a twenty year old patient with 50 percent partial thickness and flash burns. Although Bob had been on the unit for only a few days, he had already gained a reputation among the staff as an uncooperative patient. June was busily using tweezers to peel away dead skin tissue on Bob's shoulder, to allow the underlying healing tissue to surface. When the antimicrobial creams are applied to debrided areas it can be very painful. June was reminding Bob of this. She told him in a firm voice, "Now I'm not going to debride too much today because the medicine will burn too much. I'll just do a little. You'll appreciate my wisdom on this and I don't want to hear you bitching all afternoon. That's why I'm doing just a little at a time."

At nursing report early one morning, Jessica, one of the evening-shift nurses was explaining to the other nurses the problem she had that night with Chuck Thomas, a young male with 65 percent body surface burns. "Last night he kept crying and begging me not to turn him in bed. He sounded so pathetic! After he did this several times I told him, 'Chuck, please give me a break. I can't stand that begging! You know I have to do this to you, so don't beg. It really gets to me and I feel terrible.' Well, then he started saying he's sorry." Gwenn, one of the other nurses grinned at her, "And that makes you feel worse, right?"

Patients also learned very early in their stay that they couldn't use their discomfort as an excuse for not doing things for themselves. Each patient had to achieve some level of independence, no matter how painful.

Britt McCarthy was a twenty-five year old electrical worker who sustained severe electrical burns to his arms and chest when he came into direct contact with high voltage wires. The day following his admission he asked his nurse Maureen to position his television set so he could see it better. Maureen shook her head, "Move it yourself Britt; you still have your arms. What you don't use, you lose. Move the T.V. yourself." Britt complained, "But I can't move my arms!" Maureen moved closer to the side of his bed and looked at him, "Listen to me Britt. I know your arms are burned, but you can use them. Today we're going to make you feed yourself too, to see how you do."

While in general patients learned the appropriate ways of responding to and accepting pain, there were a few instances when a patient's tolerance of pain was viewed by her/his nurse as almost heroic and such patients often were given small rewards for their efforts. George Dunbar, in his sixties, and critically ill during several points in this hospital stay, had just gone through an especially difficult and painful dressing change and hadn't complained much beyond his usual level. His nurse Vera, had changed all of his dressings by herself, because the rest of the nursing staff was too busy to help, so that she particularly appreciated George's cooperation that day. The dressing change took well over an hour. When Vera was finished she smiled at George, "You've been real good George; is there anything you want?" George replied quietly, "Yes, I would really love a Coke, you know that?" Vera turned to me and whispered, "Well, he's only supposed to have clear liquids, but as far as I'm concerned right now, Coke is a clear liquid!"

To sum up briefly, nurses and therapists attempted by various means to define the reality and meaning of pain sensations for patients. Patients, in turn, learned how their pain was connected to the recovery process and thus realized their most difficult lesson: "Only in pain will you heal." Likewise patients learned the appropriate responses to pain, the various norms that defined the conditions in which certain pain expressions would be tolerated and condoned. Moreover, patients came to realize that they would have to accept their pain and working through their discomfort, carry out those activities of daily living considered crucial by staff to their recovery.

The four coping strategies I've just presented in this section all had to do with ways that the burn unit staff employed to structure the pain experiences of burn patients. Due to a number of considerations, foremost, that the use of large amounts of morphine was not in keeping with the burn unit philosophy, staff had to rely on other non-pharmacological means to help patients come to terms with their pain. As we have just seen, these strategies were a blend of social and even psychological devices that in some way forced patients to control, take charge of and better understand their pain. Each of these strategies, however, were derived from not only the needs of the patient, but, just as importantly, the needs of the staff to control their work, maintain the structure and integrity of the burn care setting and to come to terms with their own doubts and ambiguities in doing pain work.

The Response Effect

Before turning to a discussion of pain trajectories and how this concept can help us understand work in a burn unit, I want to give brief attention to some observations made in connection with the use of pain medications on the adult unit.

While the use of morphine was restricted on this unit, staff did try a variety of oral pain medications on patients. These pain medications varied with respect to strength and duration of relief; each type had unique pharmacological properties and different drugs would have success with different patients. Surgery residents and nurses were familiar with a number of pain medications and while a few types were the most frequently used, they were by no means the only medications tried.

As patients progressed past the emergent phase of recovery and staff felt confident that a full recovery would take place, morphine injections were discontinued, and oral pain medications were substituted. Many patients had medical orders that allowed nurses to administer morphine "as needed," but most nurses chose not to unless there were unusual circumstances. The oral pain medications used

most frequently had varying combinations of codiene and phena-
cetin, and it was these types of medication that nurses used in their
pain contracts with patients. Most of the nursing staff tended to
agree that while patients responded differently to these various
drugs, none of the medicines were sufficiently strong or effective to
eliminate the kind of pain that burn patients had to endure. Yet,
during the course of this study a curious phenomenon began to occur in regard to the use of the oral medications.

Patients often asked their nurses if it was possible to change their
pain medication to obtain greater relief. Many patients weren't
aware that there were other types of drugs available and thus were
quite pleased when they learned from nurses that indeed various
kinds of medications could be tried. The nurses in turn would ask
the attending surgeon for changes in a patient's medication and most
often the residents would go along with the request even to the point
of inquiring of the nurse what he/she would suggest.

When the new orders were written, nurses informed the patient
that she/he was now beginning switched to a different type of pain
medication. Subsequently, patients almost without exception, reported to the nurses that they were getting greater pain relief from
the new drug. And this added relief would usually continue for at
least several days.

In fact, however, and as the nurses and surgeons were themselves
aware, these new orders called for medicines that pharmacologically
were not stronger than the medication the patient had been receiving all along. Granted that body chemistries are different and subtle
changes in types of drugs might produce different effects in patients,
I feel that what was really taking place here was the "response effect."
What the patients were responding to was not so much the chemical
properties of the new medication, but the validation of their pain experiences by nurses. Since pain was such a difficult fact of life for
burn patients, and given that much of their emotional and mental
energies were spent in dealing with pain and trying to overcome it,
their pain experiences became almost overwhelming. While nurses
validated that patients were indeed in pain and would continue to be
in pain, it was also important for patients to believe that the nurses
were concerned enough to help them get some measure of relief. Patients had to be reassured that their complaints about their pain were

real and worth doing something about.

In the response effect, patients were reacting to the nurses' recognition and validation of what was to them very real and cause for concern. Patients began to feel better in the very act of nurses responding to them and giving attention to their requests for changes in pain medication. As sociologists have known for a long time, when a situation is defined as real, it has real consequences. This well-worn sociological proposition has no better support than in the response effect. While pharmacologically many of these patients should have felt no differently with the switch in medications, the fact that they said they were better meant that their definition of reality was based on something other than the drug itself. What this implies for pain control on a burn unit is that patients' pain alleviation was as much due to the social and psychological characteristics of the setting as it was effected by the chemical properties of the drugs that were used. Put differently, the physiological effect of pain-relieving drugs was heavily influenced by the interactions between patients and care givers. The act of responding to and validating a patient's needs and concerns about pain determined how the patient subsequently perceived the effectiveness of pain medications.

Pain Trajectories

In burn recovery, the medical and nursing staff not only constructed dying and recovery trajectories, they also put together pain trajectories, or stages of pain experiences and related problems that staff expected all patients to undergo. Pain trajectories like all trajectories were a means of organizing work and activities in the burn unit as they gave staff a way of managing and predicting patients' pain experiences. The trajectories were formed around staff expectations that patients would undergo varying levels of pain and accompanying problems throughout their hospital recovery period. Pain trajectories had contour and duration; they had a beginning phase, a middle stage and a close, which corresponded to the emergent, the acute and the rehabilitative stages of patients recovery from burns. Let's turn our attention now to each of the phases that shape the pain trajectory.

The beginning of the pain trajectory was marked by the inital assessments by nursing and therapy staffs about how well each newly admitted patient would handle their present and anticipated pain experiences. While making these inital assessments, the staff looked for clues as to the patients' past histories of pain, and how well each patient was coping with pain even on the first day or earliest hours on the burn unit. Since therapists and nurses wanted patients to "work through" their pain, this willingness or capacity was among the earliest clues searched for by staff as they interacted with patients in the first few hours.

Leon Johnson, twenty-seven years old, had been burned while working on his car, and was brought to the burn unit, by ambulance, with 20 percent burns to his shoulders and arms. He was conscious upon arrival and soon found himself submerged in the hydrotherapy tank as members of the burn team began to clean and debride his wounds. Joan, the physical therapist on duty, was dabbing at some of the burned areas on Leon's shoulder and she encouraged him to talk, though he was shy and appeared frightened at first. Joan coaxed him, "Are you married Leon?" He nodded weakly, "Yes, my wife came with me in the ambulance." Joan responded, "That's good. How many kids do you have?" "We have two boys," Leon answered. Joan continued her probe, "Well, I bet they keep you pretty busy. Leon, in your work do you get a lot of cuts and bruises and things like that? Have you ever been hurt?" Leon managed a shy grin, "No, not really. Actually I'm kind of a baby about those things." Joan laughed and reassured him, "Well don't worry, most people are like that!"

Joan continued prodding Leon about his reactions to being injured, and all this was her way of predicting how well Leon would do as a burn patient. Occasionally patients gave a staff a pleasant surprise, by showing a marked willingness to endure pain even as they were first admitted to the burn unit.

Gary, a twenty-three year old male, was undergoing hydrotherapy on his second day of admission. He had sustained acute burns of 40 percent to his arms and chest, and Joan, the therapist, expected Gary to have a difficult time in his first hydrotherapy session. Gary was well built and muscular, and he rested silently in the water the entire time it took Joan to scrub his burn wounds. He wouldn't talk to her and often shut his eyes and winced, but never once groaned, screamed or asked Joan to stop. When Joan was finally finished, she took me aside where Gary couldn't hear and said, "Boy, that's what you call a high pain threshold! He never made a peep and that had to hurt awfully bad." Joan decided to put Gary through some stretching exercises which he did without complaint and Joan continued to be impressed as she looked over to me and winked several times. She had many words of encouragement for Gary and told him when she had finished, "Gary, you're really going to do well in here. You just keep that up."

While initial assessments in the beginning of the pain trajectory were important, they could be misleading in deciding how a patient will tolerate pain later in the recovery process. This was partly due to the fact that most patients were receiving morphine injections during their first few days and this did relieve them of much of their pain. Also, many patients were still in psychological as well as physical shock from their burns and as a result, didn't respond to much of any stimuli, whether painful or not. And, of course, some patients were unconscious upon arrival and thus it was days before staff could have any idea about how such patients would respond to pain.

The more crucial aspect of the pain trajectory and the point at which staff expected patients to experience their greatest pain and related problems was not so much in the beginning, but during the middle of the recovery trajectory or the acute phase. This was expected for several reasons. One, during the middle weeks of recovery patients were fully conscious and required to make daily trips to the tank room for debridement and dressing changes. Two, in the actue phase patients' skin was beginning to heal and close in, and, as we discussed earlier, this was usually painful. An finally, it was in the middle weeks of recovery that patients began to develop anxieties about their status as burned people. They were now becoming aware of the problems associated with identity change. For these reasons, among others, staff expected the middle weeks of recovery to present the most significant difficulties in helping patients deal with pain.

Myra, the physical therapist on duty that day was complaining to some of the nurses in the lounge about Ned Rice, a thirty-nine year old patient who was in his third week post-burn. "You know I'm concerned about Ned because he doesn't work through his pain. He's been here three weeks now and he just won't give that extra effort. He cooperates and doesn't complain while he's in the tank, but he won't work through pain on his exercises. He gives up too easily! And he's in for a lot more pain and a rough road as far as his recovery goes."

During the acute phase and middle of the pain trajectory, patients began to get reputations among staff as complainers, especially those patients who were failing to live up to the terms of the pain contract and demanded increasing amounts of pain medication. Patients began to fear their daily dressing changes, the exercise periods and the other painful things they had to submit to in their daily physical care. While nurses anticipated a certain amount of patient manipulation and uncooperative behavior in this phase, there were tolerance limits that defined how much patients could get away with. When patients exceeded these limits, nurses became frustrated and exasperated.

Shortly following nursing report, as the evening-shift nurses were starting their tour of duty, Sheri, one of the day nurses, reported to them about Eric, a twenty-year old male, who was quickly developing a reputation as a complainer. During his first week on the unit he tolerated pain fairly well, but now Sheri informed the group, such was not the case, "Eric is getting to be such a cry baby. He can't take anything now. He cried and screamed all week-end long and he keeps asking for pain meds all the time. Every time he saw me today he was asking for pain pills."

Patients too realized at this point that each new stage of their recovery brought new procedures or physical changes in their healing that almost always were accompanied by different kinds of pain. Ollie, who was over sixty years old, and who had been on the unit for several months told me one evening, "You know Jim, just when I get a little bit comfortable and find a day of relief from my pain, somebody comes into my room with something new for me to do, and it always hurts!"

The final phases of the pain trajectory corresponded with the rehabilitative stage of physical recovery, the last week or two of a patient's stay on the burn unit. At this point, a patient's wounds were mostly healed, and there was increasing talk among staff about releasing the patient back to home and family. For many patients surgery had covered much of their full-thickness wounds and their pain was subsiding to a certain degree. However, joints and muscles were stiff, and the new skin usually brought itching sensations that most patients found very uncomfortable. Moreover, at this point, patients were fitted with pressure garments which were placed over healing wounds to reduce scarring and disfiguration and imporve the skin's subsequent appearance. Pressure garments were fitted a few days prior to a patient's release from the hospital and patients were required to wear these tight-fitting garments for twenty-four hours a day, up to two years. The garments were painful to put on and take off and often during the process, healed areas of skin would break open and patients would develop new sores.

Thus even at the end of the trajectory new types of pain and discomfort emerged for patients, although, in part, these discomforts were mitigated by the fact that patients were looking forward to going home and returning to some normal relationships and activities. Burn unit staff helped patients at this point by continuing the use of pain and anti-itching medications and through giving patients detailed instructions about how they could care for their healing skin when they were discharged from the hospital. For those patients who never tolerated their pain very well while they were hospitalized this final phase signaled a degree of relief for nurses and therapists who were anxious to see these patients leave the unit and return home. In some instances both patients and staff reached an impasse in their pain work, in which the patient lost all pain tolerance and staff lost all their sympathy and good-will toward the patient.

As we look at this phenomenon more closely, for a few patients, the final stage of the pain trajectory and rehabilitative phase heralded their most painful period and experiences. Despite the fact that for these patients their wounds were mostly healed, and, in a physical sense, they were nearing the time when they could return home, their ability to tolerate the remaining pain seemed to have vanished. For these patients, whatever coping mechanisms they developed in the initial and middle phases of their pain trajectory and recovery periods now failed them completely in the final weeks or days before they were to leave the unit.

Such was the case of Kelley Taylor, a young woman who had burned herself severely in a suicide attempt. Kelley had sustained partial and full thickness burns to her arms, face, neck and hands which required numerous surgeries during her two months as a patient on the unit. As a patient, Kelley never had an easy time with her pain, but in the final days her pain sensations and expressions intensified greatly much to the dismay of her nurses and fellow patients.

One afternoon I was sitting in the television lounge with Eric and while we were chatting, Kelley was having parts of her dressings changed while in bed in her room just down the hall from the lounge. At first she was moaning loudly but soon the moans changed to yelling, shouting and uncontrollable sobbing. Kelley's cries penetrated almost the entire burn unit and Eric and I could hear her quite clearly. I asked Eric, "I guess Kelley's having a rough time." Eric nodded, "Yeah, she's been like that the last day or so. I try not to listen to it because it kind of gets me upset and almost half sick. I don't know why they can't give her something."

Later I asked Maureen, Kelley's nurse, about the ordeal that afternoon. Marueen explained, "There's just no medicine except a lot of morphine that can handle that pain. Kelley worked with a hypnotist for awhile and it did help. She tries self-hypnosis on the dressing changes, but it doesn't seem to work now. She's just lost all her tolerance. Nothing we do seems to help and she's got nothing left to give her self."

Kelley was discharged home the following week and normally when a patient had been on the unit as long as she had there would have been a little send-off and an occasion made by the staff of her leaving. This did not happen with Kelley, who left quietly and almost unnoticed with a few members of her family.

While the pain trajectories were a way of organizing meaning and pain experiences, and a way of giving predictability to pain work and problems, as we have seen, trajectories were subject to variability. Most patient trajectories tended to peak in the middle of the recovery period where pain problems were most numerous and severe, and usually leveled off in the rehabilitation phase near hospital discharge. For some patients, however, there were not peaks or valleys, but a continuous series of painful episodes that never seemed to lessen in intensity and for which no coping mechanisms were very effective.

In these instances, nurses and therapists tried a variety of means to help these patients, from recommending hypnosis, relaxation-therapy, medication changes and the like. When nothing appeared to work, there remained little to do for patient and staff, but hope the time would quickly come when the patient could go home.

Staff-Conflict: Unresolved Issues

Thus far in this chapter I have presented in some detail the pain work of burn unit nurses and therapists, but have said little of the activities of the surgery residents. The reasons for this is because the residents were rarely confronted with the problem of patients' pain. With the exception of early morning rounds when they saw patients who were still half asleep or when they were called in to examine a new admission, residents didn't spend much time on the unit and had little to do with the daily physical care of patients. Though the surgery residents were the medical authority and in that sense responsible for the recovery of patients, this usually took the form of writing medical orders, that the rest of the team carried out. Whatever problems that developed as a result of patients' pain were primarily to be dealt with by nurses and therapists.

Nurses relied on the surgeons to write pain medication orders and in this endeavor, most residents wrote orders consistent with what the nurses felt appropriate to manage a patient's pain. When changes were asked for, the residents normally were accommodating to nurses' suggestions. Conflicts between surgeons and nurses in the area of pain control were not as much a conflict of orders, but rather, centered around surgical and medical decisions of the residents that nurses felt would increase patient pain and thus make their work more difficult and stressful. Conflict also arose on those occasions when surgeons interfered with how nurses felt pain medications should be administered. I would like to close this chapter on pain work by looking at these conflicts in more detail.

Nurses confronted their work with burn patients with expectations that the work would proceed smoothly and routinely, with a minimum of upset and problems. Especially in the area of pain work, nurses tried to minimize the extent to which they had to inflict pain and were concerned that, in carrying out their procedures of daily care they didn't cause patients to have more pain than was absolutely necessary.

While nurses could exercise some control over their own work schedules it was sometimes the case, that decisions by residents disrupted the orderly flow of nursing work and in turn increased the likelihood of producing extra pain for patients to endure.

One area where such problems occurred with some frequency had to do with patient dressing changes. Often in the course of a dressing change, surgeons wanted to examine patients when their dressings were totally removed and the wounds cleaned so they could check the progress of wound healing and make decisions about the necessity of surgical grafts. Normally this worked smoothly as nurses would inform the resident when a particular patient would be "open" and the resident would arrange her/his schedule to be there at that time to inspect the wounds. On occasions, however, residents failed to appear at the appointed time and the nurses had to keep the patients open for several additional minutes waiting for them. This waiting period increased patients' pain and discomfort because their burned skin was exposed to the air that much longer which irritated the skin and intensified pain. Patients would begin to complain about their discomfort and usually blamed the nurses for their situation.

A variation of this problem happened one morning and I was informed of it by Myra, a physical therapist. "You should have been here yesterday Jim; it was really something. They brought in a young guy with 90 percent burns. We had him back in the tank room for over three hours cleaning him up and getting his dressings on. It took four nurses to help because he was burned so bad, and he was in such pain we wanted to hurry and get him covered up. Well, after we were all finished, McGregor (Surgery Chief) called and said he wanted to see him open! So we had to do it all over again!"

Decisions made by the residents while in surgery about the types of dressings used to cover grafts and donor sites also made the work of nurses more difficult. This was especially true if the type of dressing laid on in surgery caused pain for patients when nurses subsequently worked with them in giving daily care.

Earlier I introduced Kelley, a young woman burned in a suicide attempt. During one of her skin graft surgeries, the residents had left her fresh donor sites open, except for some gauze wrapped around them, instead of putting on the synthetic protective dressing that was normally used. When the nurses discovered this after surgery, they applied an antimicrobial cream to the donors to prevent them from becoming infected. A few days later when the nurses began to un-wrap the donor site dressings to check the healing progress they real-ized that the creams had adhered to the raw skin. In removing the dressings then, Kelley was in severe pain. Glenda, her nurse, re-marked to me, "I don't know why they (residents) didn't put the reg-ular dressings on Kelley's donors. Especially someone like her who has lost all her pain tolerance."

Also, surgeons' decisions about which antimicrobial creams to use on burn wounds have implications for nurses' work because some of the topical creams tend to irritate burned skin more than others. When surgeons decided to change their orders on a patient's topical dressings from one that the patient was tolerating fairly well to another type that nurses knew would increase the patient's dis-comfort, the nurses realized that their work with that patient would become more difficult.

This was demonstrated one day in the children's unit in the case of a fourteen year old girl, Maggie, who was burned badly on her chest in a house fire. None of the topical dressings used on her burns were promoting wound healing or decreasing infection, though sur-geons tried a number of different types. After several days, the chief resident suggested to the nurses that they switch to a topical dressing known to be effective in such cases, but, also considered very painful when used on children in the past. Kristie, who was Maggie's nurse that day, told the resident, "O.K. If we are going to use that topical on her, then you are going to have to take her surgery on every dressing change and put her out. We won't be ale to handle her! Maggie can't take the topicals we've been using without throwing a fit, and it takes three nurses to hold her when we do her dressings as it is now!" With reluctance the surgeon agreed to use the operating room for her dressing changes.

Conflict between nurses and surgeons also surfaced when pa-tients appealed to the residents for extra pain medication in violation of the pain contract, and also, on those occasions in which surgeons interfered with nursing judgments about pain management for par-ticular patients. Surgeons could, of course, prescribe or order pain medication for patients at their discretion, while nurses could only administer medications as ordered. Patients knew this, and often talked the residents into changing their medication orders or increasing their allotments, even though the nurse might have felt that what was already being done for the patient was appropriate or adequate. As this happened, nurses considered that the agreements about pain medication that they already negotiated with patients were now being superceded by residents, who changed the orders at a patient's request. Nurses were particularly upset when residents acted upon a patient's request and were not familiar with the patients circumstances and current condition.

The importance of the medication conflict was pointed out to me by Gina, one of the nurses on the adult unit. Gina recalled, "I was taking care of Millie the other day and she had orders for morphine "as needed." Well I had just given her two milligrams of morphine for her pain, but I was afraid to give her any more because her respirations were so low. Morphine tends to depress a patient's respirations anyway. So when Millie asked for more I said "No." Well, later in walked Dr. Grey to examine Millie and Millie told her that she was in a lot of pain. As Grey walked out of the room she said to Millie, 'Your nurse will give you something for it.' But Grey never said a word to me! Now how does that make me look with the patient when Grey tells her something like that?"

Such misunderstandings between surgery residents and nursing and therapy staffs occurred with some regularity on both adult and children's units. While breakdowns in communication between levels of staff are typical in every hospital setting, in the burn unit they were especially awkward and disconcerting for nurses who were committed to the team concept and, relative to the surgeons, held less power. Moreover, with respect to pain work, decisions by residents that increased and made nursing work more difficult not only frustrated them and added to nursing stress, but, at times, worsened the pain experiences of patients. As the latter occurred, patients tended to hold accountable and vent their displeasure toward those persons who were most familiar, accessible, and vulnerable, the members of the nursing staff.

Chapter Five

THE COMPLIANCE PROBLEM IN BURN
RECOVERY

IN the nurses' lounge, a few minutes past the noon hour, I was sitting with Susan and Vera, two of the nurses on duty that day, and
as the morning had been very busy we were glad for the change to sit
down. Vera had dished up two plates of salad from a large plastic
bowl that Susan earlier had taken from the refrigerator. I sipped on a
soft drink as the two nurses started in on their salads. Within moments we looked up to see Gwenn, one of the other nurses walk into
the lounge carrying a medication chart. Gwenn claimed one of the
empty chairs and as she sat down, she remarked to Susan, "George
told me an interesting thing about you today, Susan." Susan put her
fork down and smiled, "Now what is he saying?" Gwenn replied,
"Well he said you were so busy this morning that you were ineffi-
cient. You're not taking good care of him." Susan was no longer smiling, "You know Gwenn, I've heard just about enough out of George.
As soon as visiting hours are over, I'm going to have a little talk with
him! I'm getting tired of this!" Gwenn and Vera laughed at Susan's
display of temper, and quickly changed the topic of conversation as
they continued their lunch.

Around two that afternoon I followed Susan into George's room
where he was resting in bed looking uncomfortable. George Dunbar
was in his sixties and had been burned severely when gasoline ignited as he worked in the garage of his home. George had suffered
partial thickness burns on nearly 50 percent of his body including

large areas of his chest, back and arms. This was George's third week post burn and he had been subject to infections throughout much of his hospitalization. The residents were having a difficult time getting him physically stabilized to the point that he could undergo surgery. As Susan entered his room, she said to him. "George, what is this you've been telling Gwenn? I've been really busy today, but I've still given you good care!" George acted surprised at the confrontation and answered weakly, "Oh, I know it Susan. I'm not complaining. Except that I asked you for a drink of water and you didn't give it to me." Susan responded, "That' not exactly right and you know it George. You asked me for a Coke and I said you could have a sugar-free soft drink. You're not supposed to have much sugar George!" Looking sheepish and defeated, George said quietly, "Well I guess I must have been confused." Susan turned to leave the room, "I guess you were."

At George's request, I remained in the room a few minutes longer. George stared in my direction, "It looks like I've been told." I laughed at him, "You sure were George." He looked annoyed now and squirmed in his bed, "Oh, she's just out of sorts with me. That's nothing new. And now she'll be like this with me all day."

The following morning, George Dunbar was again the topic of conversation of Vera, Susan and Gwenn who were working together in the nurses' station busily writing information in patients' calorie charts and medication records. Vera was bothered that George continued to be so demanding, "The thing about George that really gets me is that he wants us to feed him his meals. Doesn't he ever learn? He's got to feed himself and we're just not going to do it for him." Susan nodded in agreement, "Yes, and he wants to be in bed all the time too. But I'm not going to let him do it. He has to be up in a chair for a certain amount of time, especially for his meals." Gwenn looked up from her chart and asked Vera, "Who is down there in the room with him now?" Vera replied, "Oh, that's his girl friend and his sister. Whenever they're here they wait on him hand and foot. About every five minutes they come up here asking for something that George needs."

Late in the afternoon of that same day I was on rounds with Joel Horling, the plastic surgery resident and Adam Friedman, the resident in general surgery. Both men had been in the operating room most of the day and it wasn't until nearly five o'clock that they were able to make rounds in the burn unit. They were still dressed in their green surgical scrub suits. Horling and Friedman moved methodically from room to room intently checking over the critical care flow sheets that were posted outside each patient's room.

As we walked into George Dunbar's room, George raised his head off the mattress and started in on Joel Harling, "Now doctor, you just can't keep me flat on my back like this. I want to be able to sit up in bed. It hurts me to be flat in bed; I've got a bad back you know." Horling moved slowly to one side of George's bed as Friedman sat on a nearby stool and continued to study the medical charts with George's most recent laboratory studies. Joel leaned over the side rails of the bed looking at George, and said in a tired voice, "Now what's the problem here George?" George began to whimper, "I just told you the problem doctor. I'll get convulsions if I lay flat on my back like this. You just can't keep me down on my back. I had surgery a few years ago!" Joel was patient, "Well part of the day you need to be flat in bed George. You've got burns around your neck and you need to be in a position to keep that skin from drawing down. Positioning is important for something like that. There's no getting around it." George got more forceful and was no longer whimpering. "I'm saying that I can't take any more of this. If you doctors can't figure out another way to treat me and make me more comfortable, then I'll just leave and go home."

At that point Adam Friedman placed the lab reports on a table and walked up to the side of George's bed opposite Joel. Horling looked in Adam's direction, smiled, and then turned back to George, "You're giving me an ultimatum now and that can't be done. No matter where else you go, I don't care what other hospital in the city, you're going to get the same treatment. If you go home you'll be a mass of scars and you won't be able to raise your arms. And I'll tell you something else George. You're not out of the woods yet. You have severe burns and you could still die." George looked stubborn, "Then I'll go home to die." Joel raised up and looking at Adam, shook his head slowly. He even shot a glance at me without saying anything. After a few moments he turned back to George, "Do you have any family?" George replied, "Yes, my son visits almost every day and my girl friend too." Joel nodded, "Well, I'll talk with them and see how they feel about this." George looked up at Horling, "Doctor, couldn't I at least sleep on my side? That would help so much." Joel agreed, "I don't see any reason you can't do that. I'll talk to your nurse about it." George started to complain, "That won't do any good. Nothing I do seems to please them." Horling pushed himself away from the bed and smiled down at George, "Well don't worry about that. Around here nobody can please the nurses."

As the three of us departed from George's room, Joel invited me for a cup of coffee in the lounge. As Joel sipped carefully from his coffee mug, our conversation soon turned to burn patients such as George Dunbar. Joel explained to me, "You know George is in his sixties and it's my experience that older persons can't take burns as well as young people. They just don't have the stamina." I responded, "George does seem to be uncomfortable a lot of the time." Joel thought for a moment, "Yes, but it's more than that. I suspect that George is the kind of guy who has been a pain-in-the-ass all his life. He's probably been a pain-in-the-ass to his family too. And now he's the same way in here."

The three-month career of George Dunbar as a patient on the adult burn unit was frequently characterized by the kind of scenes and conversations I have just presented. Many other examples could have been taken from field notes to demonstrate the point that, in the eyes of the burn unit staff, George was an uncooperative and frequently noncompliant patient. Stated differently, the sorts of attitudes and behaviors George displayed during his recovery often were contrary to the many values and demands of the burn care setting.

This chapter on compliance addresses some of the most fundamental problems in all rehabilitation and recovery programs: to what extent must patients become involved in their own recovery; and how do hospital staff see to it that patient compliance to a recovery program is brought about? The compliance problem was at the heart of much of the work of residents, nurses and therapists in this study and compliance needs to be carefully examined to have a full understanding of the general nature of burn recovery.

Burn patients were expected to participate and cooperate in their own recovery. In many ways, the burn unit staff admonished patients to "Pick Up Thy Bed and Walk." The values of the burn unit setting were such that patients could not passively lay in bed and wait for their conditions to improve. Patients had to be actively engaged in the recovery process. They were obligated to cooperate and work with the staff in directly confronting the physical and emotionally demands of the recovery/rehabilitation program. While each patient's pain was recognized and validated, and some degree of forced dependency was expected, the values of the burn unit setting required patients to assume some measure of control over their recovery.

Compliance in the burn center meant essentially that all patients accept the Recovery Program. In an interview with the head nurse on the adult unit, the recovery goals were explained, "Patients have to *want* to get better. It doesn't do any good if they walk out of the burn unit with straight arms and functional fingers, if they go home and get depressed and don't continue the program. It's the year post burn when patients develop contractures and lose mobility! We (nurses) have to instill in them that "the program" is their program. It is what they want. And that is very hard to do. If patients say to us. 'I don't want to do this, I just want to die.' you can't respond by saying, 'That's O.K. Just go ahead and die.' You have to show them you are really concerned for them. You pour yourself into them."

Acceptance of the Recovery Program signified for the staff that patients were, in an emotional sense, committed to their future. One of the nurses in the burn unit linked the Recovery Program to an emotional test of individual will-power, "One of the things burn patients must have is the will for survival. And if they have this, they must go along with the program. They have to take the calories, do their exercises and so on. If they cooperate in this they're going to do better. The uncooperative ones, well, I think they just don't do as well sometimes. But they have to have the will to want to get better."

In sociological terms, the Program referred to the routine life of the burn patient: styles of action and being expected by the staff of all patients. To comply was to accept the Program which mandated the patient to be a certain kind of person and to act in specific ways. Both requirements meant that patients had to see themselves in a new way.

No matter what patients were like before they were burned, staff expected them to be and act cooperatively, to comply with the daily regime of recovery demands and to commit themselves to their recovery. However, pre-burn personalities and behaviors often were thought to be linked to a patient's actions while on the unit. While pre-burn characteristics were not accepted as an excuse, they were considered as an explanation of present behavior.

Two of the nurses on the adult unit, Susan and Vera, were talking late one afternoon about Zack, a patient with whom the staff had continual compliance problems. Susan looked at Vera, "Zack just has no motivation at all! He just lays there all the time and he is capable of helping himself." Vera questioned her, "Well, is he retarded or what?" Susan shook her head, "I don't know, but he was like that when he came in. His family says that's the way he was as a kid. He ate his meals alone and walked all stooped over. He's been like that all along. His brothers seem fine!"

The non-compliant patients quickly developed reputations on the unit as uncooperative, and often their failure to come to terms with the setting demands was linked to suspicions of alcoholism or other personality disorders. In these cases, personality pathologies were thought to inhibit a patient's ability to adapt to the new styles of being and action expected on the unit. This occurred with Ollie, a sixty-five year old patient severely burned while smoking in bed. When Ollie was brought to the burn unit, laboratory studies revealed a high level of alcohol in his blood. This finding and other of his behaviors defined Ollie as an alcoholic and colored his reputation as a patient during his entire four-month recovery.

One morning Vera was walking Ollie to the shower for his daily dressing change. Ollie had been a patient now for over two months, but continued to find this shower and dressing changes very painful and often complained and cried throughout the process. As Vera guided Ollie into the shower room and was preparing to remove his dressings, Ollie stopped her and said, "I've got to have a bowel movement first." Vera agreed to that and while Ollie was in the toilet she turned to me and said, "He is such a procastinator! Anything to put it off." She then called out to Ollie, "Why didn't you go to the bathroom earlier?" Ollie answered, "I did! Now I've got to go again." Vera looked annoyed, "Ollie, I got you up at eight o'clock. You had time to do all of this then. You didn't eat your breakfast or take any of the pills you were supposed to!" Vera then turned back toward me and lowered her voice, "Ollie's an alcoholic and he's contankerous. He's used to getting his own way all the time."

Other nursing specialists attributed patients' lack of compliance and uncooperativeness not so much to pre-burn personalities and behaviors, but rather to the disorganizing effects that severe burn injuries have on normal personality adjustments. Here, the burn injury itself was seen as an assault on coping mechanisms that left some patients virtually helpless in adopting the behavioral and attitudinal requirements of the burn care setting. This explanation was offered by Mellisa Taylor, a nurse mental health clinician, who often was called to the burn center to counsel those patients whom staff considered especially troublesome or non-compliant. "I find that burn patients often lose all defenses and control and are reduced to basic infantile instincts. In this state, they start crying and whining for things, and, of course, the nurses have a real problem with that. But this is usually temporary and as patients improve physically they come out of it and gain some control of their actions. It's a stage that many of them go through early on. And this is when the nurses tend to invite me in for help."

While sociologically the Program called for modes of action and being considered appropriate for patients' recovery, in practical terms, action and being centered around some very specific setting demands that all patients were expected to adhere to. I would like to examine these demands in some detail.

The first requirement of the Program meant that patients were expected to do for themselves and show as much independence in activities of daily living as was physically possible. As stated earlier, some degree of forced dependence was accepted, especially in the emergent phase when patients were still critically ill and in physical and emotional shock from their burn injury. However, as patients entered the acute phase of recovery they were required to feed themselves, dress themselves, brush their teeth, walk to and from the bathroom and shower, and in similar ways become independent. Such physical accomplishments were considered important and necessary by staff to enhance range of motion, prevent muscle and joint stiffness and to normalize patients' identities. While these activities of daily living were painful for patients to endure, staff were reluctant to tolerate much complaining or whining about them. Staff took it for granted that patients would learn to do these things.

On the children's unit, Mike, an eight-year-old boy was frequently wetting his bed and forgetting to call his nurse, LuAnne, when he had to urinate. At first LuAnne was tolerant of this, because Mike earlier that day had his urine catheter removed and often this caused patients to wet themselves until they became accustomed to urinating without the aid of the catheter. But later in the day when Mike continued to have problems LuAnne had a talk with him, "Now Mike, you can't keep doing this. You're eight years old and shouldn't be wetting the bed. When you have to go, use the urinal here on your bed and ring the buzzer for me when you're finished. Now you have to do this. You're a big boy."

On the adult unit, nurses were having a problem persuading Gary, a twenty-year old patient, to get out of bed for his meals and to eat sitting up in a chair. One morning his nurse prepared a large sign and posted it outside the door to Gary's room. The sign read, "Gary Must Be Out of Bed to Eat. Put His Tray On a Stand Across From His Bed." All the nurses were warned, as was Gary, that the only way he could get his food was to walk across the room to his tray. If he insisted on staying in bed he would have to go hungry.

A second element of the Program that patients had to conform to was calorie intake. Physiologically, large amounts of calories are needed to promote wound healing, due to the fact that the human body absorbs tremendous numbers of calories in fighting the effects of burn trauma. Thus in the burn unit, eating foods high in calorie content was seen as one way patients could take direct control of the healing process. Patients were continually reminded by the staff that the more they ate the more quickly their skin would heal and the sooner they could leave the hospital. For many patients, depending on their physical size, body weight, and total surface area burned, this requirement meant that they had to consume thousands of calories per day. While some patients enjoyed eating and had hearty appetites, many patients because of their immobility, constant pain, and emotional stresses had a difficult time eating food.

For those patients unable or unwilling to maintain their daily level of calories, the staff would insert a naso-gastric feeding tube that passed through their nose into the stomach. These patients continually were fed liquids high in calorie content and there would be less emphasis given to how much they ate during their regular meals. Burn patients often developed food anxieties about their ability to eat enough food to maintain their daily required calorie level and in turn comply with the expectations of their nurses. One patient complained to the surgery resident during rounds, "Doc, I just can't eat enough to keep these nurses happy." The resident replied, "You'll never eat enough to keep the nurses happy, so don't worry about it. Just eat what you can. That's why we have you on the feeding tube anyway."

While a few patients welcomed the feeding tube as it lessened their anxieties about eating, other patients found the feeding tube uncomfortable and awkward. Nurses on both the children's unit and the adult unit used the tube as an inducement for patients to eat all the food on their trays and their between-meals snacks. "Eat or Get the Tube," was a phrase heard often from nurses in dealing with patients who continued to have problems in meeting calorie requirements. On the children's unit, when youngsters were receiving their nourishment through the feeding tube it lessened some of the troublesome aspects of their daily nursing care. Darla, one of the nurses on the children's unit remarked to me, "I'm glad Artie's (patient) on a feeding tube because now we won't have to fight with them about eating. We have enough things to fight with him about with his dressing changes and medications and everything else!"

A third dimension of the Recovery Program involved the daily physical exercises in which each patient had to participate. Exercising was essentially the domain of the physical and occupational therapists, but even the nurses enforced the exercise routines required of each patient. As we saw in an earlier chapter, physical exercise was considered important by staff to prevent contractures and maintain a patient's range of motion. Burned skin tightens and contracts especially over joints such as elbows, wrists, and shoulder areas. Without exercises to loosen the skin and keep joints limber and flexible, burn patients can develop contractures and loss of joint mobility which in turn can leave them virtually immobile and unable to lift their arms or use their hands. To prevent patients from becoming physically handicapped, every patient was put on a daily regime of physical exercise. These exercises were painful routines for patients, but, as in other aspects of their recovery, they were expected to exercise faithfully even when nurses or therapists were not present to prompt or remind them.

During an afternoon physical therapy session in the exercise room, Joan, the therapist, was working with Phil Richardson on some arm and shoulder exercises. Joan asked Phil, "Where's your buddy Gary (another patient); he should be in one these exercises too. He really needs the work." Phil answered quietly, "In his room, I guess." Joan turned to me and said laughing, "Go get Gary out of bed and tell him to get down here. Throw ice on him if you have to." A short time later Gary walked stiffly and slowly into the exercise room. "I'm really tired, couldn't I skip this today?" Joan replied, "No, you can't. You don't want to let Phil have all the fun himself do you?" As I stood next to Gary I kidded him about his beer that he was permitted to drink the night before. Phil perked up a little, "Beer? God I wish I could drink a case of it before I go to the tub. Maybe that would help." Joan asked Phil, "How much are you walking each night Phil?" "Oh, just down to the bathroom and back." Joan shook her head, "That's not enough. You need to do more Phil. I want you to walk the entire hall four times a night. And (pointing to Gary) take your buddy here with you. He needs it too."

Patients differed in their willingness to endure the exercises. Some couldn't understand the reason for the exercises and resented the intrusion of another painful ordeal. Not only did these patients dread the exercises, but they also began to resent the staff, whom they blamed for causing them unnecessary pain.

I was sitting in the television lounge with Eric, William and Tom watching an afternoon soap opera. Everyone was relaxed and quiet when Evon, one of the physical therapists walked into the room and said to William, "Come on, let's go down to the exercise room and do some work." William let out a cry, "Evon, I done my exercises already today with Sandi!" Evon said firmly, "Well you're going to get some more. Let's get going." After William left the room, Eric turned to Tom and said in a quiet voice, "Before you're through in this place, you'll hate the nurses more than you'll hate your burns."

Not all patients would have agreed with Eric's assessment. Some patients won the respect and admiration of the staff by their willingness to exercise without complaint.

Myra, a therapist was exercising George Dunbar while he lay in bed. She was putting him through some hand and wrist exercises. As she did so, she was providing instruction for Jacki, a student nurse on the burn unit. At one point she commented to Jackie, "See this area on George's shoulder where it's getting so tight? Well, often patients will need surgery to correct that, but Bobby Williams (another patient) had that same tightness in his shoulder and he exercised out of it. He exercises all the time even though it hurts him. I'm telling you, when I work with him, he wants to feel pain. He knows if it doesn't hurt it's not doing any good. When we srub him in the tank room he wants it to hurt. He might scream, but he never wants you to go easy on him."

Indeed this latter point gets at the core of the final aspect of the Recovery Program, and that is the expectation that patients will endure the painful elements of their recovery without complaint. Pain and discomfort cannot be an excuse. As I pointed out in the previous chapter, patients were required to work through their pain and go the extra mile. While brushing one's teeth with burned and blistered fingers might be agony, patients had to accept this as necessary in their recovery. A trip to the bathroom might seem like hours for patients whose stiffened and painful legs could hardly carry them. But if the staff had removed the urinal from their bed, patients had little choice in the matter. Every patient had to come to terms with the Program and no amount of complaining or begging would be to any avail.

Having looked at the nature of the Recovery Program and the importance of patients compliance, it remains now to detail just how compliance was brought about. For as one can imagine, few patients adopted the attitude of Bobby Williams and asked for more exercises. In fact, even Bobby had moments in which the staff felt he was giving up and demanding less of himself than he might. Most patients as they entered the acute phase and began to realize that they could not simply lay in bed hoping their pain would subside and that their skin would heal, gradually became cognizant of the fact that they would have to live out a life on the burn unit that was in some ways similar to the life they lead before they were burned. They came to see that in varying degrees they were expected to take charge of their own recovery and actively engage themselves physically and emotionally in their own rehabilitation. This realization, however, was essentially thrust upon them by the medical, nursing and therapy staffs. In making patients come to terms with the demands of their rehabilitation, the staff was engaging in compliance work. Getting patients to comply and cooperate with the Program was not taken for granted by staff; it was not something that staff assumed that patients would do naturally or automatically. On the contrary, experience always demonstrated that few patients would willingly take up their beds and work through their pain. Rehabilitation from burns was something that the staff had to initiate and structure for patients.

Evoking compliance, or getting patients to "buy in" to the Recovery Program was not an easy task from the burn unit staff and it constituted some of their most important social and psychological work. This work also resulted in some of the major frustrations that the staff experienced with burn patients. In the sections to follow I would like to explore the methods used by staff in their compliance work. I will analyze these compliance tasks in terms of two rather general categories of activities that I refer to as compliance socialization and developing trust. We will look at Compliance Socialization first.

Compliance Socialization

Given that relatively few patients would be familiar with and willing to adhere to the demands of burn rehabilitation, most patients had to learn what was expected of them in their recovey. Compliance socialization refers to a broad-based process of socialization in which burn patients learned their expected roles and the demands of the setting. Patients learned what they were supposed to do and the kinds of persons they were to be. This learning took place in an informal manner, in their daily interactions with residents, nurses, and therapists, who taught them the expectations of the setting. Most of the teaching was done indirectly by implication and inference, and within the context of the routine life of the burn unit. The socialization was a gradual process and involved a patient's slowly coming to terms with the demands of the setting and his/her place within it.

With respect to identity, patients were to be cooperative, self-motivating and disciplined, and ultimately their own healer. Staff expected patients to take command of their recovery destiny, to initiate some measure of control over the healing process and their physical rehabilitation. Moreover, patients were to become the kinds of persons who would do these things on their own, without complaint and reluctance. Patients learned these styles of being in the daily routines of their physical care as staff continually reminded them that only by taking charge of their own rehabilitation would they fully recover.

Sandi, the occupational therpist, was constructing an arm splint for Ned, a thirty-nine year old patient who was in his second day on the unit. Though positioning his arm from the splint caused Ned some pain, he didn't say anything and did everything that Sandi told him to do during the half hour it took to make the splint. When she was finished, Sandi patted Ned on the arm and looked directly into his heavily bandaged face, "Ned, you are a very cooperative patient, and that means a lot in here. If you keep that up it will help you a lot to get better."

Staff also reminded patients early in their hospital stay, that the staff was not only in authority on the burn unit, but were no-nonsense types who tolerated very little noncooperative behavior. Thus patients learned that the sooner they became self-motivating and self-disciplined persons, the easier the patient role would become for them. Often the nurses portrayed this tough-minded view of themselves in a humorous and kidding manner, though the message was implicit.

Bob Corona had been a patient on the burn unit for only a few days when he was in the tank room having his dressings changed by June and Wendy. June was an experienced burn nurse and Wendy was completing her orientation as a critical care nurse. Bob Corona had already earned a reputation as a patient who didn't always cooperate and June wanted to get their relationship established on the proper footing. Although June's style with patients was normally very direct and serious, on this morning she took a teasing approach with Bob. As she began to cut away at his dressings, she said to him, "You know I'm a mean nurse. I'm just plain mean and that's why Wendy is working with me today, so she can take lessons in meanness from me. In fact, Bob, we're going to be so mean to you that you'll want to get well in a hurry and get out of here!"

Referring to the above case, while Bob Corona's behavior had been contrary to the norms and expectations on the unit, it was too early in his stay for staff to confront his behavior directly. Thus, for at least the first several days, nurses and therapists kidded him a good deal, hoping he would get the message in that way. A few days later, however, when Bob was refusing to eat more than just small portions of his food the staff got more forceful with him. One morning as he was sitting in the television lounge smoking a cigarette, Peg, the physical therapist and his nurse, Vera, entered the room and asked him what he was doing. Bob answered them, "I'm having a cigarette." Vera looked at him, "Well, you haven't finished your breakfast." Bob nodded, "I'm not that hungry. I didn't sleep well last night." Vera walked across the room and disconnected the television, "Bob, you get back to your room and finish your breakfast. No television until everything is eaten." As Bob started down the hall, Peg called to him in a stern voice, "Don't you know the nurses will give you the tube if you don't eat? You don't want that do you? Now Bob, you need food to heal, so let's eat that breakfast."

Burn patients also learned from staff that they were to be the kind of person who would accept their pain and discomfort as routine events. Even during their first few days on the unit, the staff pulled patients out of their silence and quiet suffering and into the web of sociability on the unit. Patients were taught that suffering was routine and unavoidable and that they were to make the most of the circumstances and carry out their lives on he burn unit as normally as possible.

Duke Young was fifty years old, a large and powerfully built man; he was burned severely in a fire aboard his fishing boat. His neck, face and shoulders were burned badly but he had not sustained an inhalation injury and was able to talk. However, on his first day on the unit he barely uttered a word and lay silently and unmoving the entire day. Early the following morning, Myra, the therapist and Gwenn one of the day-shift nurses went into his room and got him out of bed, onto a cart and wheeled him to the tank room. Duke's face and lips were swollen and he remained silent, but Myra talked to him continuously. "You're a big man Duke. How tall are you?" Duke didn't answer and kept his eyes tightly shut. Myra continued, "I said how tall are you Duke?" After a few moments

Duke whispered through his swollen and cracked lips, "About six feet one." Myra replied, "Well, that's pretty tall. I understand you like boats. What kind of boat do you have?" Again Duke lay silently on the cart with his eyes closed and he was softly moaning. As Myra and Gwenn began unwrapping his dressings, Myra prodded him, "What kind of boat do you have, Duke?" Duke sighed deeply, "A fishing boat." Gwenn responded, "Oh, can you take people water skiing? We love to ski. Can you ski behind your boat?" Duke kept his eyes shut and between his moans he answered, "Not on that boat." This went of for several minutes as Gwenn and Myra continued to prepare Duke for hyrdrotherapy. Each time Duke tried to avoid answering a question and remain silent, Myra would open up a new line of conversation. To each question Duke had to respond. After several more minutes, when Duke was finally ready to be lowered into the water, Myra gave him some instructions. "Now Duke, today we're just going to clean your wounds, but tomorrow you will have to do exercises in the tank. You can just lay here today, but tomorrow we start to work. O.K.?" For the rest of the hydrotherapy session Duke was allowed his silence, which was only interrupted by his moans of "Oh, God. Oh, God!" as Gwenn and Myra began to clean his wounds.

During the initial period of socialization as patients learned to be cooperative and self-motivating, they often were excused from their failures to live up to staff expectations. However, patients were also made to realize that these failures would not be tolerated indefinitely and that once the early grace period was over they would be on their own and expected to live up to standards.

Maureen was taking a breakfast order one afternoon from Britt McCarthy, a young male with acute electrical burns to his arms and chest. Britt had put in an order for bacon and toast. Maureen looked at Britt and said, "Do you know that you are supposed to get 4200 calories a day? Your toast and bacon are only about 200 calories Britt, and that's just not enough." Britt responded, "I just feel so awful; I don't know if I can eat any more than that for breakfast." Maureen nodded to him, "Well, 200 calories isn't enough, but we'll let it go for today." Later that afternoon, Wendy a student nurse who was assisting Maureen with Britt's care, walked ito the nursing station where Maureen was sitting, "I'm trying to get Britt to feed himself, but his arms and hands are so awkward he keeps spilling things. I'm afraid he'll spill something on his fresh bandages." Maureen agreed, "Wendy, it's probably too early to push him very hard. Britt is still in the edema stage and suffering from the trauma of his injury. But I do think he needs to feed himself, but let's give him one more day."

Once beyond the first week or two of their recovery, burn patients were expected to know their routines and obligations so well that they were to be completely self disciplined. With respect to their daily rehabilitation, patients were required to know what was correct and proper, and make necessary adjustments.

Ollie was in his second-month post burn and because of burns to his arms and shoulders, he was been fitted for splints on his arms to hold them in positions that would prevent contractures. These splints often would slip into improper positioning and since Ollie was familiar with his program he was expected to re-position the splints to the correct angles. Ollie rarely remembered to do this however, as he found the proper positioning physically uncomfortable. One afternoon, Sandi the occupational therapist, came into Ollie's room to give him some exercises. When she spotted his splint positions she became visibly upset, "Ollie, what are you doing? Look at your splint!" Ollie acted annoyed at her displeasure, "Why, what's the matter?" Sandi moved to the side of his bed, "That's not the correct position! And you know better than that Ollie. It's not doing you any good positioned like that."

Likewise, in later stages of socialization, patients were admonished to do and to know not only what was correct in terms of their daily care, but to continually endure their pain and affirm life as a positive value. Burn patients were taught to believe in themselves no matter how difficult their recovery was, how bleak their future appeared, or how painful their daily care was proving to be.

Several nurses in the staff lounge were discussing the situation of Britt McCarthy, a young man in his twenties with severe electrical burns. Britt's arms were so badly injured that the surgeons were considering amputation. In addition, he was experiencing acute pain because of the burn-induced swelling of his lower extremities. Maureen put her coffee cup on the table and told the other nurses, "Well he's at his sickest now. He is so edemous and it's very painful. His testicles are all swollen up and he doesn't want anything painful done to him. Now he even refuses to have blood drawn." Vickie asked Maureen, "Well what did you tell him about that?" Maureen replied, "I told him, 'Britt, we have to draw blood. You are a very sick man. Do you want to die?' Then he said he didn't care if he died or not." Vickie shook her head, "He's no picnic to work with. He gets mad at us whenever we do anything to him. He doesn't want to be awakened in the morning. He wants to smoke in bed, and he can't do that. What a mess!"

In addition to the identity expectations and socialization into self-discipline and self-motivation, patients were also taught the norms of compliance. More to the point, patients learned that the nurses were in charge and their directives were authoritative. Compliance in the burn unit meant above all that nursing rules could not be challenged and that in nearly all aspects of their daily recovery care, patients were to look to the nurses for approval. Ideally, patients were expected to do what was correct in promoting and quickening their recovery, in practical terms, however, doing right was engaging in those actions that satisfied the nursing staff and generated their approval. This point, above all else, was learned by patients very early in their burn unit career.

Maureen was applying fresh dressings on the burn wounds of Britt McCarthy the morning of his second day of admission. As she was putting the finishing touches on the dressings, Britt murmured, "That's enough tape." Maureen smiled at him and said good-naturedly, "Sounds like you're calling the shots around here. Well, I like my dressings on tight, so they won't fall off while you're in bed." A few minutes later as Maureen was positioning pillows under and around Britt's legs and arms, he remarked that the pillows weren't comfortable. Maureen looked at him and said, "This is the way you are supposed to be positioned, Britt. And that's the way it is. And by the way, after today I call the shots."

While patients learned many things about their recovery in terms of compliance, including that the nurses were in charge, they also learned they could expect little sympathy for their plights and situations from the staff. While nurses and therapists often expressed in their private conversations that they felt badly for a particular patient, such attitudes or feelings were rarely displayed directly to the patient. In fact, patients found that the nursing and therapy staffs seldom gave in to or allowed attitudes of resignation or defeat to be talked about. When patients were doing poorly, they were expected to improve their performance, and if they were doing well, there remained an extra measure of attainment that the staff would look for.

Myra, a therapist, was in George Dunbar's room exercising his arms and hands. George was cooperating and working hard although he complained several times how uncomfortable he was. Myra stopped after about ten minutes and said to him, "Well that's good George, but we'll try to do more." George looked over at me and said with a touch of annoyance, "Oh sure, that's all you ever hear around here." Later in the evening I was chatting with George while he lay in bed and he was complaining that the nurses wouldn't feed him. "They make me feed myself and my hands are all wrapped up and so sore I can hardly stand it. I tell you Jim, I love these kids (nurses) and they work so hard. But sympathy is what they have the least of." As George made those remarks, I was reminded of a statement made a few weeks earlier by Val Gorham, a patient who had been on the unit for over a month. When referring to the nurses and therapists he said, "You know, words of discouragement are something you never hear around this place."

Patients were also socialized into compliance on those occasions when nurses and therapists presented them with a grim vision of a dark future. Those patients who were reluctant to wear continually their position splints, or those with neck burns who refused to lay flat on the mattress and insisted on sleepng with pillows got reminders from the staff about the disfigurements and contractures that would develop in their future. Therapists often informed patients that daily exercises and position splints were the only means of preventing future surgery that would be needed to correct contracture deformities. Here was a variation of the "Eat or you get the tube." Now patients were admonished to "Exercise or you'll have to return for surgery." For those patients who continually defied their therapists and avoided exercising on their own, the staff would evoke compliance by showing them pictures of burn patients with severe neck and hand deformities. These graphic displays were accompanied by verbal warnings from the staff, "Is this what you want to look like two years from now? With your chin pulled down to your chest?" Patients normally responded with a sense of dismay and promises to work harder and with more regularity.

Other times therapists and nurses would encourage patients through more positive reinforcers. When some patients got discouraged with the exercises and lost sight of recovery goals, they would be introduced to more fully rehabilitated patients who had similar physical problems. On a few occasions this involved visiting a patient on another ward who had successfully prevented deformities through rigorous exercises and use of position splints. During clinic days, when former patients visited the hospital to have their at-home recovery monitored, they often returned to the burn unit to encourage patients there to stay with the Program. Certain celebrated patients who had survived massive burns were used by the staff as models of compliance for other patients to emulate. Patients currently on the unit were challenged by the staff that if these former patients could survive devastating injuries and lead physically normal lives, surely they could do the same. In these cases, the vision of a dark future was contrasted with the image of a bright or at least normal future for those patients willing to comply with the exercise routines.

Compliance socialization was accomplished also through the use of small bargaining agreements between patients and staff as means of rewarding patients or giving them a measure of control over their care. Bargains were trade-offs in which patients were induced to live up to the requirements of the Program in return for some minor reward or favor from the nurses or therapists. Most of these agreements were temporary, informal, and even spur-of-the-moment decisions by staff. Nevertheless, in the routine life of the burn unit, they occurred with frequency and proved somewhat successful for staff in gaining compliance. While the bargains might not ensure a patient's total commitment to the Program, they might work in getting a patient to accomplish something on a given afternoon.

Since eating and exercising were two activities most burn patients had difficulty with, the bargains were more frequently used there. Maureen, for example, had been struggling for several days to persuade Danny Horton to eat more food. Danny was on a 4400 per day calorie requirement but his usual in-take fell far below that. This afternoon, after Maureen saw that his lunch tray had barely been touched she said to him, "Danny, you've got to eat more or you're going to get the tube again. And I know you don't want that. Do you like junk food?" Danny looked puzzled, "What do you mean?" Maureen replied, "Things like hamburgers, French Fries or potato chips. Will you eat that?" Danny agreed, "Well that would be better than the stuff they give me here." Maureen looked encouraged, "Alright, we'll try to get you some food that you like. And you better eat that!"

In a similar vein, eating was used as an inducement to other rewards or favors that some patients sought, such as permission to return to bed after exercise therapy. Late one afternoon I was in the television lounge with Danny Jones playing a video-bowling game with him. The video game was the idea of the therapists who felt that was a good way to get Danny to use his arms and hands that were badly burned in a car accident. At this point in his recovery Danny didn't like to be out of bed for very long because of his pain, and he had been in the television lounge for nearly an hour. From his wheelchair he continued to call for his nurse, Maureen, to get her permission to go back to bed. Finally Maureen appeared in the doorway of the lounge and asked him how long he had been up. Danny replied, "I've been in here for over an hour, haven't I Jim?" I agreed. Maureen nodded, "O.K. That's good Danny. You can go back to bed, but first I want you to brush your teeth and drink a milk shake. You're still 500 calories behind today. Will you do that?" Danny said he would. Maureen started out of the room, "Now which flavor of shake do you want? It's up to you."

Likewise exercise sessions which patients rarely could avoid occasionally involved small choices for patients that induced them to participate with some degree of enthusiasm. Joan was in Gary O'Neil's room to give him his afternoon exercises. Gary wanted to lay on his back for this work, but Joan informed him, "You can't lay down Gary. You have to sit up. But you can do them sitting up in your chair or on the side of the bed. You can choose; either one is fine with me." Joan went on to explain why the exercises were necessary for his recovery.

Bargains over compliance even reached the minutia of physical activity. Patients who were being persuaded to feed themselves at meal time were told by nurses that if they would agree to use their hands to hold the fork, the nurses would cut up the food on their trays.

Such agreements were also employed on the children's unit. This was especially the case in efforts to get children to eat, which was a major compliance problem in the Recovery Program for the children. Meeting their daily calorie requirements proved a difficult undertaking for most of the children in this study.

Megan was a twelve-year old girl who was burned in a propane explosion during a family camping trip. After she was successfully fluid resuscitated and taken off intravenous feedings, the nurses had a difficult time in getting her to eat. Paul, one of the nurses on the children's unit tried some bargaining with her to increase the amount of food she would be willing to eat. One day after lunch Paul said to her, "Megan, you've just got to start eating Hon. Food makes you heal. You've got a bad burn and it's not going to get better if you don't start eating more. Would you like to do something special today?" Megan responded very quietly and shyly, "Like what?" Paul smiled at her, "Oh, I thought we could make some flags to decorate your room. If we made enough we could put flags up all over the unit. How does that sound?" Megan agreed. Paul then told her, "Well, you've got to eat first. No food, no flags." Megan protested, "But I'm full!" Paul examined her plate closely, "Full? You can't be full; you only ate three bites of bacon! Now listen, I can be a mean nurse if I have to. You probably never saw a male nurse before did you?" Megan said quietly, "No." Paul grinned at her, "Well I can be a meany. So eat some more on that plate and we'll make some flags this afternoon, O.K.?"

Later that same day during nursing report, one of the other nurses, Julie, asked Paul if he had any success in getting Megan to eat. Paul laughed, "Well, I'm getting there I think. Of course what I didn't tell her is that we have ways of dealing with children who don't eat." Julie smiled and said, "Yes, they get the tube!"

Developing Trust

A bond of trust between staff and patients was considered by staff as crucial to promote compliance. Nurses and therapists felt that patients were more likely to accept the demands of the Recovery Program if they trusted the staff to do what was right. If patients thought that the therapists and nurses were acting in their behalf, then they would be more likely to work through their pain and comply with the program. Given this point of view, staff sought ways to gain a patient's trust and acceptance. Put more directly, the staff tried to show concern and care for their patients as a mechanism for establishing that trust.

Among the ways that trust was accomplished in the burn units was through personalizing relations with patients. From their first day of admission, patients were referred to by their first names or nicknames and this informality characterized interpersonal relations in the burn care setting. Staff went to some lengths to learn about the personal lives of their patients: their birthdays, anniversaries, family circumstances, their jobs, hobbies, interests, favorite foods, and so on. In turn, the staff quite willingly shared with patients this kind of information about themselves. During painful dressing changes and hydrotherapy sessions, nurses and therapists would draw patients out in conversation about their lives and activities outside the hospital. Once a nurse or therapist learned some details concerning a patient's personal or social background, this knowledge was used as a basis for talking, joking or kidding while performing the daily routines of patient care.

In a more general sense, on both burn units, sociability and intimate interaction replaced the more formal and impersonal staff/patient relationships. On the adult unit, for example, most of the patients were male and the nurses and therapists were female. Trust here was established and maintained through a type of role-distancing, in which informal, cultural male/female teasing and joking often replaced the more formal nurse/patient roles. To a certain degree, some of the culturally defined roles between men and women, which in hospital settings are usually obviated by the professional-client model, were allowed to carry over into the adult burn unit interactions. Interpersonal trust was accomplished, in part, by de-emphasizing the kind of social distance that accompanies formal client-professional role relations.

Burn unit nurses and therapists wanted to be accepted by their patients. This was partly because acceptance formed the basis of trust, but also acceptance made the work of the staff more agreeable and tolerable. Therapists and nurses expected their patients to be friendly and sociable with them just as they were toward the patients. Thus there was a norm of "effortless sociability," which required that the daily routines of patient care would be carried out in a context and mood of friendliness and sociability. Interpersonal relations were quickly upgraded on the burn unit, so that within a few days of a patient's admission she/he was made to feel an intimate part of the world and well anchored in a matrix of relationships with staff and other patients.

In addition to sociability and the upgrading of personal relationships, trust was also established by staff through showing concern for patients. Staff often devoted considerable energy in demonstrating their concern for a particular patient. Occasionally such activities involved the violation of hospital rules, but, according to one of the most experienced burn nurses I talked to, all of this was part of good nursing. "You have to pour yourself into your patients. You show that you care for them by doing a lot of little things. Fix their hair up before visiting hours; bake a cake for their birthday; let their kids visit incognito. Put some cologne on them. Act weird! Anything that will work. As nurses we see these burn patients at their worse moment, but you still care about them and think they are worthwhile people. When I used to work with children sometimes we would sneak a puppy into the burn unit. To that child, that is therapeutic. If it makes the patient feel better then that's nursing!"

Establishing a sense of interpersonal intimacy with patients was not always easy for staff. As we have seen, many patients wanted to take to their beds and suffer alone and in silence. Rarely, however, were they permitted to do that.

The less-experienced nurses frequently were frustrated when they were unable to "get through" to a patient and gain some degree of acceptance. On the children's unit one morning, Sarah, a recent nursing graduate was lamenting that she was having a problem with her patients, two young girls burned in a family camping trip. Sarah told Julie, one of the most experienced nurses, of her frustration, "You know the Evert girls just aren't reacting to us (nurses) at all yet. They just demand things, but they won't talk to us or anything!" Julie nodded, "Yes, I know. But that's to be expected the first few days. Pretty soon they're going to warm up to you. Just go easy on them right now, Sarah. Go into their room every so often and do things for them and they'll get to know you."

Another way nurses showed concern for patients was through acting as advocates in their behalf. For example, when patients expressed a desire to change to a different pain medication, or asked for permission to have their children visit the unit, or requested some other special privilege, nurses often would present their case to the senior resident or medical director. Patients often trusted their nurses to help them secure privileges that they could not gain on their own. Even surgical decisions provided opportunities for nurses to intercede for those patients with whom nurses felt especially close.

Glenda had been Bobby Williams' nurse for several consecutive days. Bobby had been on the unit for over a month with 90 percent body surface burns. His condition had now stabilitized to the point that the surgeons could begin a series of skin grafts. The day prior to his surgery, Glenda approached Adam Freidman, the general surgery resident, who was sitting in the nurses station, "Adam, how much are you going to try to get grafted on Bobby tomorrow?" Adam looked up at her, "Well, we're going to do as much of his legs as we can." Glenda nodded, "Do you think you could get to his butt and graft some of that? He can take the pain in his legs if only his butt wouldn't hurt him so." Adam smiled, "We'll have to see; we want to get his legs first, and if we can do more, we'll try to get that for him."

To summarize briefly, patients compliance was accomplished not only through a process of patient socialization and learning, coupled with the small bargaining agreements between staff and patients, but, also by the ways in which staff attempted to show care and concern for their patients. By demonstrating concern for patients, staff hoped to win their acceptance and trust, so that patients would feel part of the social world of the burn unit and thus become more willing participants in their recovery care. Concern, acceptance and trust emerged out of the daily interpersonal relations between staff and patients which emphasized a certain degree of shared intimacy, close interpersonal bonds and upgrading of social relationships intended to make patients feel "at home." These primary-like relations between patients and staff were also a means of redefining some of the negative and disagreeable aspectes of pain work performed by therapists and nurses. By seeing themselves as friends and intimates with their patients, staff were better able to come to terms with their role as pain-inflicters.

Pushing

Despite these manifold and varied ways used by staff to induce and gain patient compliance, not all burn patients worked to their potential or met the demands of their individual recovery program. This was due, in part, to the fact that some patients' personalities and methods of coping simply prohibited them from working through their pain. For other patients their burn injuries were so severe and complicted that their recovery demands were far above what the patient could normally deal with.

These cases called for what staff often referred to as "pushing." Pushing meant that the staff had to employ extra measures of efforts to prod or challenge a patient to go beyond what they were initially willing to do. To a certain degree, many nurses and therapists felt that nearly all burn patients needed to be pushed to do more in their rehabilitation than they would do on their own. However, other staff felt that some patients needed pushing more than others. Let's look at this phenomenon more closely.

The philosophy that all burn patients need some degree of pushing, was explained in an interview I had with Donna, one of the senior nurses on the adult unit. Donna viewed pushing in this way. "All patients need to be pushed. It's pretty rare that a burn patient is self-motivated. It just hurts too much. But you can't let the patient choose the therapy. Ninety percent of burn patients don't want to hurt themselves. That's why we (nurses) take off their dressings. It's too painful for patients to do it themselves. A patient can be angry at the nurse, because she's the one that hurts you. And I think that's O.K. But hopefully, they look back and say, 'If the nurses hadn't made me do this I wouldn't be able to straighten my arm.' You hope that light dawns on them that way."

The place and importance of pushing in burn recovery was further elaborated on in an interview I conducted with Sheri, a woman with many years of burn nursing. "Pushing involves our getting patients to take more calories, to do their exercises, and to do more for themselves. As many things for themselves as they can possibly do. Now, I see pushing as encouraging patients. Patients just cannot lay back in bed and sleep to forget their pain. They need to be encouraged to be up and doing things to help themselves get better. And one of the ways you encourage patients is to work with them more. If you (nurse) have some free time, get the patient out of bed and do some exercises with them."

I asked Sheri why it was so important that patients be pushed or treated so aggressively. She answered, "Well it's the goal to get the patients out of the hopsital more quickly, isn't it? The harder patients work the faster they will get out and return to normal. It's better therapeutically to get them home where they'll feel better about themselves."

Elaine, a physical therapist who had worked with burn patients at several burn centers in the United States felt that pushing was at the core of burn rehabilitation. "Burn patients in general have more potential than they push themselves to. And I won't set limits on them. If someone without fingers says 'I can never type again,' I would say, 'You can if you want to.' Because you can type with your mouth or arms. Burn patients need to feel that they have some power over their destiny. And this is the therapist's job."

In the routine line of the burn unit pushing was manifested in the many ways staff prodded patients to do more in their recovery. As Sheri pointed out during our interview, in practical terms it meant asking patients to eat more food, exercise a bit longer than they did the day before, sit up in a chair for increasing periods of the day and so on. For patients, pushing meant that one small effort on their part lead to the staff asking them for still more.

George Dunbar had been confined to bed for several weeks because of severe infections, but on this particular day, he had improved enough to be able to have a hydrotherapy session in the tank room. After an hour in the tank room and with his fresh dressings in place, Myra, the physical therapist, talked George into taking a few steps from the dressing cart to his wheel chair. George was shaky and feeble but he managed three steps on his own and sat in the chair. Myra was quite pleased. "Oh George, that's just great! Now later this afternoon after you take you nap we're going to get you walking down the hall a little!"

Families of patients often were seen as allies of the staff in the pushing efforts. They were encouraged by staff to persuade their wives or husbands to go the extra mile in hastening the recovery process. One Thursday in Team Conference on the adult unit, Phil Richardson's case was being discussed. Burned over 50 percent of his body, Phil had been hospitalized nearly a month. Maureen, one of the nurses attending Conference that day described Phil, "He's doing better, but he needs to be pushed. But his wife Irene is good. I talked to her and she thinks Phil needs to do more for himself. She told him that she is not going to let him rely on her for everything."

Patients tended to differ in terms of their reactions to pushing. Some patients got very angry and frustrated, rather than encouraged. I was with George Dunbar one afternoon in his room during visiting hours. He was sitting up in a chair talking to his son, whom he wanted me to meet. George told us, "I don't like sitting up in this chair because it hurts my back! Jim, I've done all they ask of me. I eat and I take my medicines and wear my splints. All I want is to be in bed. Why can't I have that? What more do they want of me?"

However, other patients came to realize that only by being pushed did they recover or make significant progress. Often this realization came some time later in a patient's recovery career. Tim Wickers was a patient on the burn unit for several weeks to have reconstructive surgery on his face. The previous summer, Tim had been burned in an electrical accident at work, and in addition to losing both arms through amputation his face was badly burned and disfigured. Tim and I were talking about his experiences in the television lounge one morning and he remarked, "Jim, when I was in here for three months last summer, boy the nurses and therapists used to really push me hard. And I would get mad. I just wanted them to leave me alone. But now, I realize it was for my own good. I wouldn't be here today if they didn't push me so hard."

On the children's unit, most of the pushing was concentrated at meal times in getting children to eat all their food. Both staff and parents alike prodded and coaxed the children to eat as much as they could. Although with children, the nursing staff recognized the limitations of pushing during meal times. As Julie, one of the nurses explained to me, "It's so difficult to get the kids to eat and take those calories, but not eating is the kids' only means of controlling their situation. They can't refuse their tubbings or dressing changes, they have to take their medications and naps, but they can always refuse to eat! That is their control of what for them is a pretty tough situation. So we're leary about pushing them too hard, because they might get to the point where they won't do anything!

Thus pushing had its liabilities and limitations in the burn units. Few patients, during the short run, willingly accepted the relentlessness of the staff in getting them to do more and go beyond what they thought was comfortable. As was pointed out earlier, most patients did not want to invite more pain and discomfort than they already had. Nevertheless, nearly all therapists and nurses saw it as their responsibility to continually ask for more than patients were willing to give. While their relationships with patients were open, friendly, encouraging, and at times intimate, the staff always pulled back at a certain point and disconnected themselves long enough to demand that the patient reach a higher level in his/her rehabilitation. If recovery from burns was thought to be a never-ending battle, then the nurses and therapists were the aggressors, and few patients were allowed to remain aloof from the hostilities.

Clinic Days

I would like to close this chapter on compliance work by looking briefly at burn clinic and its relation to the compliance problem in general and at-home recovery specifically.

Upon being discharged from the hospital, most burn patients were neither completely healed nor entirely physically rehabilitated. However, many patients had been hospitalized for such an extended time, that the burn unit staff felt there would be emotional and psychological benefits if patients could be at home for the final stages of their recovery. Patients were discharged with the understanding that they would return to hospital clinic once each week to give surgeons and therapists an opportunity to monitor their recovery progress and correct any problems that they might be experiencing. Aside from being responsible for doing their daily dressing changes and skin care at home, patients were instructed by the therapists in the various daily physical exercises they were to do. Each patient received pamphlets and charts detailing the required exercises to improve range of motion and increase the functioning of their burned limbs. The at-home recovery was basically an extension of the Recovery Program started for the patient during their stay in the burn unit.

On the clinic days then, therapists and surgeons examined a number of patients who were at various stages of their at-home recovery. Some patients would be returning after having been home a week, while other patients were over a year post discharge. Surgeons checked these patients for progress of wound healing, signs of infection and to determine surgery needs to correct disfigurations or enhance range of motion. Patients with contractures, who were unable to lift their arms or bend their fingers would be scheduled for release surgery, which was a procedure to loosen or release tightened skin.

Physical and occupational therapists examined clinic patients for range of motion and to assess how well they were carrying out activities for daily living. Therapists were also anxious to determine whether patients were complying with the exercise regime, and if they were faithfully wearing their pressure garments to reduce scarring. During the examinations, patients would be asked to raise their arms, make fists, grab onto objects, etc., to demonstrate the extent of progress in their rehabilitation.

Clinic days were occasions when patients could either proudly show-off, or be ashamed of their lack of accomplishments. Either condition depended to a considerable extent on how well each patient was adhering to their Program while at home. Those patients sufficiently motivated to continue rigorous daily exercises, who faithfully wore their position splints and pressure garments and who strove to be independent in activities of daily living were usually those who drew words of praise and kind remarks from the staff. They were anxious to demonstrate their improving physical status.

Aaron Michels was just such a patient. He was a teacher, in his forties, and burned on his face, neck and hands in a laboratory explosion. While a patient on the burn unit, Aaron was a favorite of the staff because he complied with most of the demands of his Program and after he was discharged home he continued the compliant pattern.

Aaron appeared to welcome clinic days because he not only had the opportunity to question his surgeons about his progress, he also had the chance to show the staff how he was living to the very letter of his at-home recovery. On one of his clinic visits Sandi was looking at Aaron's facial scars. Sandi voiced her obvious pleasure, "Oh this looks good Aaron; these grafts are really flattening out." Aaron beamed, "Well I wear my pressure mask all the time. I never take it off. And I have been doing my exercises too. Look how strong I can grip. Come on, grab my hand." Sandi took Aaron's hand in a handshake grip and Aaron began to squeeze tightly. "How's that? Pretty good, huh?" Sandi nodded in agreement, "That's just amazing, Aaron, You've really gotten strong!" Aaron then proudly stuck out his thumb and began wiggling it around to show Sandi his range of motion, when Dr. Williams, the medical director, walked into the examining room. Aaron looked in his direction, "Hello, I'm just showing Sandi here how well I'm doing." Dr. Williams grinned, "Yes, I can see." Aaron continued, "Well, I do all the exercises that Joan and Sandi gave me, plus a lot more. I do a lot of housework and gardening. Anything to use my hands and arms. I guess it's paying off now, isn't it?" This went on for some time as Sandi and Dr. Williams stood patiently but quite pleased as Aaron continued his list of accomplishments.

At the opposite end of the compliance pole, were those patients such as Buddy Bowles whose at-home rehabilitation program was all but forgotten during the months after he was discharged from the burn unit. Buddy had been burned nearly a year earlier in a gas explosion in his home. Burned over 50 percent of his body, his face, neck, arms and hands required extensive grafts. At twenty-five years old, Buddy was a shy and unassuming young man, whose wife, Maria, did much of his talking for him. Buddy was unable to return to work because of the injuries to his hands, and he and Maria spent most of their time watching television in the living room of their home.

On one of Buddy's clinic appointments he was showing his facial scars to Joan, the physical therapist, who shook her head in disappointment with what she saw. "Buddy, are you wearing your pressure mask?" Buddy answered quietly, "No, not much. It hurts my jaw and teeth and I can't eat good when I have it on." Joan instructed him, "You bring your mask in the next time you come to clinic, Buddy, and we'll see if it needs refitting. Your face doesn't look good at all." Joan turned to Maria and pointed to areas along Buddy's chin and cheeks, "You see how this is all purple and bumpy along here? Well, it's going to stay that way if Buddy doesn't wear his mask." Buddy indicated to Joan some features of his forehead that he thought were improving. Joan responded, "Yes, but those other areas on your chin are getting worse and your face will stay purple if you don't wear your mask. Your hands look good though." Buddy proudly showed Joan his thumb release which had been done in surgery a few weeks earlier, "I think that I'll be able to make a fist now."

While Buddy and Maria sat in the examining room waiting for the medical director to begin Buddy's examination, Betty, the unit social worker took me into the hall outside the room. "Dr. Williams is going to hit the ceiling when he sees Buddy's face. It looks awful compared to last month! Buddy hasn't been doing the mouth and lip exercises that Williams gave him to do and now his mouth is drawing in. You can hardly see his lips! Williams will be furious with him."

The case of Buddy Bowles was not atypical, many patients found that the pressure garments and masks were very uncomfortable when worn continually. Patients also discovered that, in public, the pressure garments drew as many stares and inquiring looks from people as did their discolored, burned skin. In fact, on a subsequent clinic vist, Buddy and Maria told an emotional story of how the police in their town came to the house one evening to question Buddy about the robbery of a neighborhood service station. Apparently the robber was wearing a mask, and since neighbors had seen a young man wearing a mask on their block, Buddy became a suspect. Months later Buddy remained disturbed by the incident, as he told Dr. Williams, "I think I would rather have scars, then go out in public and have people think I'm a criminal!"

Chapter Six

THE DYING PATIENT: PROBLEMS IN TRAJECTORY

DURING a busy Tuesday evening in the City Hospital emergency room, sixteen month old Melody Lewis was brought in by ambulance for scald burns. One of the physicians who examined her, Dr. Edward Dill, could see that much of her body was burned, but it appeared to him that the burns were superficial. He wrote orders for Melody to be admitted to the Pediatric Unit of City Hospital. Shortly after Melody's arrival in the Pediatric Unit, several of the nurses on that service suspected that she was becoming very sick and that the burns were much more severe and complicated than at first realized. On March 18, that same evening, Melody was quickly transferred to the children's unit of the Burn Center.

Very early the following morning Kristie Day and Paul Ames, two nurses on the children's unit, took Melody to one of the tub rooms to clean her wounds and begin a dressing change. Meldody was wide awake and very fussy. As Paul and Kristie began to slowly and carefully peel away the outer surfaces of Meldody's dead skin they immediately discovered that nearly all her burns were rapidly converting to third degree, or full-thickness burns. Melody had been burned to the deepest layers of her skin on over 40 percent of her body. Paul left the tub room and put in a call to Dr. Coyner, Chief of Surgery, and told him of Melody's condition. Dr. Coyner decided to put Melody on the surgery schedule for later that same morning.

Melody was operated on some six hours after being admitted,

and during surgery Dr. Coyner saw that Meldoy's arms and legs had been burned circumferentially so that as her skin began to swell and tighten, it threatened to cut off her blood circulation. Dr. Coyner made long slits in the burned skin, called escharotomies, which opened the tightening skin and relieved the pressure. Since Melody was burned on much of her arms, chest and stomach, Dr. Coyner had to place her intravenous lines for fluid resuscitation in her forehead and scalp. Melody received two IV lines, plus a catheter was inserted into her bladder to collect her urine for monitoring. A nasogastric tube was placed through her nose into the stomach to prevent her from choking on any stomach contents. She was also connected to a cardiac monitor to measure and record her heart rhythms and blood pressures. Melody's wounds were very dark and cherry red. Parts of her chest and abdomen were covered with large wet blisters. After several hours in surgery Melody was taken back to the burn unit and placed in the critical care room.

Two days later, during Team Conference, Kristie Day described Meldoy's case for the surgery resident, the physical and occupational therapists, the dietician, and two mental health clinicians. Via, the unit's social worker, was absent that day. Kristie read from Melody's file, "Melody Lewis was admitted two days ago. She is sixteen months old and has 40 percent second and third degree scald burns. Records show that she was a 'failure to thrive baby' when she was born. Dad is twenty-one years old, but not married to Mom. Dad put Melody into the bath tub for her bath and when he returned later she was face down in the tub. Mom called the ambulance." Rose, the dietician asked Kristie, "Has a child abuse report been filed?" Kristie nodded, "Yes, I guess Dad's been arrested before, but he seems so nice."

On March 25, seven days later, Melody was taken to surgery where the surgery resident grafted most of her right leg. Since Melody's back was not burned, the surgeons used that skin for donor material. Melody had no serious trouble during the two-hour surgery, although the plastic surgery resident, Dr. Landon, told the burn unit nurses not to give Melody any morphine since anesthesiology had a few problems.

On the afternoon following her surgery, Melody's mother, Lorraine, called the burn unit to inquire about her condition. The nurse who took the call, Judi, told me later over coffee, that Lorraine was pretty confused about Melody's situation. "Melody's mom seems kind of flaky. The dad seems O.K., but they just don't know what to ask. Lorraine was asking me if Melody would have scars and when she'll be able to walk. My God Jim, Melody's lucky to be alive! We're not worried about scars at this point!"

Two days after her initial surgery Melody was holding her own according to Arlene, who served as Melody's nurse that day. "She is doing a lot of fussing and crying. In fact last night I don't think she slept any; she just cried all night long. I tried rocking her to sleep and that didn't help. We gave her medications for her itching and pain, but nothing seems to help though. She was just so restless."

March 30th, twelve days following her admission to the burn unit Melody appeared to be in a crisis. Laboratory cultures of her blood samples showed indication of sepis or infection. Despite all the efforts of the burn unit staff, Melody's body temperature was falling rapidly and steadily, a sign of severe infection. About mid-morning of that day, I asked Barb, one of the nurses on duty, what she felt was the problem. Barb answered, "Melody's just not doing anything. I'm not sure if she'll make it or not."

Kristie and Barb put in place a large, electrically monitored heat lamp over Melody's bed in an effort to elevate her temperature. As a precaution, Kristie also taped a code medication card to the wall of Melody's room. She explained this procedure to me, "In case she codes (heart stops) this afternoon, we'll know what drugs to push to revive her." I asked Kristie, "You don't think she's going to code, do you?" Kristie shook her head, "With Melody you never know. But if she does, I want that code card handy. It's just a precaution."

An hour after the heat lamp had been turned on, Kristie walked into Melody's room to see the effect on her temperature. As she looked up at the heart monitor, Kristie said in a discouraged voice, "Oh, that's just great. Now her temperature is down to 30.8. We're going in the wrong direction! I give up; I'm going home."

Kristie's last remark was made in jest, for she was on hand when Dr. Coyner, Chief of Surgery, and Dr. Landon, the plastic surgery resident, came into Melody's room a short time later as they were making rounds. Moments earlier, Kristie had removed most of Melody's dressings so that Landon and Coyner could examine her open wounds. Both surgeons were wearing their surgical scrub suits and donned masks and gloves as they entered the room. Melody was awake and she cried softly at first as the two men began their examination. Much of her burns were covered with cadaver skin as a temporary graft until Melody could harvest enough of her own skin for donors. As Dr. Coyner began to peel off sections of her cadaver skin to check the burn wounds underneath, Melody began to scream in a dry, hoarse, shrieking voice that caused her body to shake. Melody was tiny for sixteen months and her thin and frail arms were secured to the sides of the bed to prevent her from picking a the grafts on her wound.

After Coyner peeled away more of the cadaver skin, Dr. Landon used a scalpel to cut a small piece of Melody's burned skin to send to the laboratory where it could be tested for infection. As he did so, Coyner turned to Kristie and said, "Let's change her topicals (antimicrobial agents) and see if that won't help her. Something's causing her to be infected and what we're using now just isn't getting it." Kristie nodded in agreement and as she was talking with Dr. Coyner she placed a pacifier in Melody's mouth and gently and slowly rubbed Melody's forehead with her gloved hand. Melody responded and began to quiet down.

Moments later Coyner left the room and sat in a nearby chair crossing his legs. As I pulled up a chair next to him, he look at me and sighed, "Well, I still think she has been worse. She's septic there's no doubt about that, but changing the topicals might get her straightened out." I asked him, "So you are optimistic at this point?" Coyner ran his hand thriugh his sandy-brown hair, "Let's say I'm cautious. I told Melody's father on her first day of surgery that she might die. And nothing has changed. But there is no obvious reason for her going down-hill now."

Twenty-four hours later, with the change in topical dressings, Melody's temperature began to return to normal. Several of the staff expressed how relieved they were that Melody appeared to be out of crisis.

Melody's physical condition remained stable and with little change for another nine days. However, on April ninth, Arlene Miller, Melody's nurse that day, told the staff during nursing report that Melody's burns looked terrible. "Especially her grafts. They not only

look bad but they are starting to smell. I know they are infected."
Sarah, another nurse on duty, told Arlene, "Well, Melody's mom
called again and asked how she was breathing. She doesn't understand what is going on at all." Arlene looked at her in agreement, "I
know. And by the way the police are going to be here tomorrow to
video tape Melody's dressing change. I guess it will be used as court
evidence for child abuse. Someone told me that the police suspect
that both mom and dad were responsible for Melody's burns."

Three days following, Melody was taken again to surgery to have
additional areas of her legs and chest grafted. Surgeons reported that
she went through this procedure with no major difficulty. This event
marked Melody's twenty-fourth day of hospitalization and it was her
third surgery.

On April seventeenth, during Team Conference, Via Simms, the
burn unit social worker, informed the burn care team about the continuing police investigation of Melody Lewis' accident. "The detec-
tive called me today and they feel that there is enough evidence to
sustain a charge of child abuse in Melody's case. So as of today, Melody's sister and brother have been placed in a foster home." Via's remarks were followed by a general discussion among the team about
Melody's home life and background. Arlene Miller, Melody's nurse
that day, pointed out to the group that while Melody's mother did
not visit every day, she called quite often to see how she was doing.
Arlene continued, "And her dad visits on occasion and appears concerned about Melody's future."

When Team Conference was concluded and the room emptied
out, Paul and Arlene remained and sat down for coffee. I asked Paul
about Melody's progress since her last surgery a few days earlier.
Paul shook his head slowly, "Well, not too good. Only 40 percent of
her grafts took. The rest of the grafts they put on just fell off." Paul
leaned forward out of his chair to hand me the pictures they had taken that morning of Melody's burns. "You can see these pictures look
awful. She still has all these areas open. We just can't get them covered." As I looked at the pictures, I saw that much of her burn
wounds appeared red and raw; some of the areas of the lower section
of her abdomen were wet and glistened. Melody still had a urine
catheter in place, and three intravenous lines in her scalp and forehead. Arlene told Paul, "Well, Melody is healing in on a few places.

And her nutritional intake is O.K." I turned to Arlene, "Then you feel she is going to do O.K., Arlene?" Putting her coffee cup on the table, Arlene leaned back in the chair, "I quit predicting on Melody. I don't know what she is going to do." After a few moments, Paul added, "Well, I never in all my experience saw a kid reject grafts totally like she does."

Dr. Coyner came in to see Melody two days later. He was accompanied by a medical student and Mary Eason, the new resident in plastic surgery. Kristie, Melody's nurse, was busily removing the dressings, so that Coyner and Eason could get a good look at Melody's burns. Within minutes Coyner turned to Krisite, "When did she last have surgery?" Kristie answered, "I think its' been about ten days." Dr. Coyner nodded and looked at Eason, "Why don't you take her to surgery tomorrow and clean up some more on her hands and toes. We need to get the eschar off there. Don't you agree, Kristie?" Kristie agreed, "It probably wouldn't be a bad idea." Melody had her fourth operation the following day.

During the surgery Dr. Eason was able to remove the burned tissue from Melody's toes and fingers. The procedure went well and Melody didn't lose any fingers or toes as some of the staff feared she might. Later that evening Lorraine, Melody's mother, visited her in the burn unit and read quietly to her from the Bible. Melody rested comfortably. Lorraine informed Arlene Miller that she was now attending a counseling center to get some help. She hoped the court would allow her other children to return home before too long.

Later in the week, during Team Conference, Kristie reported to the group that Melody was showing some subtle signs of improvement, "Melody just seems more awake and alert now. You can ask her questions and she'll nod yes or no. And she doesn't cry when people come into her room." One of the mental health clinicians asked, "But could that be due to loss of affect? Maybe she is just oblivious to everything now. Maybe she doesn't care." Kristie replied, "It could be, but I think Melody is getting used to us now and feels more comfortable having people around."

On the forty-first day of Melody's admission to the burn unit, she was placed on a special nourishment program of fluids administered intravenously. It was hoped that this extra protein would help her burn wounds heal more quickly and completely than they were up to that point. Melody continued to be restless and her nurses noted that she squirmed a good deal in her bed. Consequently, she was given several medications to help her rest more and sleep more soundly.

Earlier in the day, the physical therapist told Dr. Mary Eason that she was concerned about Melody's fingers, "I think her fingers might get worse and I doubt that they will get much better. Her fingers are curled down into a fist, except her first finger which is out. I can't seem to get them positioned right. Her toes don't look good either." Dr. Eason nodded in agreement, "I know, we probably should have pinned them when we had her in surgery last time. She needs some other areas grafted too, but I don't think she is ready for any more grafts right now."

During the morning of May first, I asked Julie, one of the nurses, how she felt Melody was doing. Julie responded, "Well, she's not going up or down. She seems to be on a kind of plateau. At this point I would say that anything can still happen. She continues to lose blood and she has hardly any healthy tissue. But her blood cultures are looking O.K. She doesn't seem to be growing anything in her blood."

As Julie was talking, Dr. Eason came in to make rounds and she sat down to talk with us. Eason pushed back some strands of hair from her forehead and leaned forward in her chair, "I just feel that Melody's going to do better. For one thing, she has eaten now for three straight days. That's real good. And I think her burns look better. To me, they just look like they are starting to heal a little."

A while after my conversation with Julie and Dr. Eason, I went into Melody's room; we were alone. I had planned to leave town for several days on vacation so I wanted to spend a few minutes with Melody. She lay quietly in her bed, on her back as she had been now for well over forty days. Sucking gently on a pacifier, her eyes were wide open and she knew I was in the room. Melody's room was somewhat dark because it was nap time on the unit. I looked down at Melody and asked her, "Would you like me to read you a story, Melody?" She nodded her head slowly up and down. "How about this one, A Book About Dogs? Would you like that?" Again she nodded, and I read to her quietly for about twenty minutes and then left her room so she could nap.

I returned from my trip four days later and visited the burn unit to check on Melody's progress. As I was putting on a yellow cover-gown over my clothes I noticed that Melody's room was empty and had been thoroughly cleaned. Turning to Sarah, one of the nurses sitting at the nurses station, I asked, "Sarah, what did you do with Melody? Did she change rooms?" Sarah stood up and looked at me, "Melody has angel wings now, Jim. She died yesterday."

That afternoon I had the opportunity to talk to Dr. Eason as she made rounds I asked her how Melody had died. Eason sat down in a nearby chair. "Well, let's see. You left on Thursday, didn't you? Well, on Friday her blood count kept dropping so we transfused her. Then she was probably septic over the week-end and we just didn't know it. On Monday we transfused her again. A chest x-ray showed pneumonia. On Tuesday she was bleeding into her right lung. We changed her antibiotics. Nothing did any good. She just went right out." After my conversation with Dr. Eason, I found Paul, Arlene and Julie who were with Melody the day she died. It was Paul's first code. Julie told me, "Melody had positive blood cultures on Monday which indicated infection and that hinders blood coagulation. She was bleeding into her lungs and this is how she died." Arlene added, "Her organs were just worn out. The body can take only so much stress. This is what burns do to people." Julie commented, "Well, we did all we could. We pushed every single drug on the code cart and every line was wide open. But nothing did any good." I asked Arlene Miller if Lorraine, Melody's mother, was able to be there. "That was interesting. At first no one could find her, so the police were sent out to look for her. Lorraine got here about five minutes before Melody died. Her dad was here too. He just sat in a chair holding his head. He was just so shocked by it all."

In this chapter I intend to focus on the dying patient in the burn unit and how the staff came to terms. The dying patients presented a number of problems for the burn unit staff, some of which were evident in the case of Melody Lewis. Melody was severely burned and her recovery was continually hampered by the fact that she was a "failure to thrive baby," and to begin with, was not physically healthy or robust. She was not well prepared physically to respond to a major burn injury. Despite this, however, Melody did not die quickly nor did she linger. Her dying career, or trajectory, was characterized by highs and lows and periods where she appeared to be holding her own and capable of recovery. As the case study illustrated, there were several points when the staff felt that Melody was in crisis and that her condition was deteriorating, yet, these junctures were followed by periods of improvement and more positive signs. Such situations nearly always gave the staff reason to take hope for a complete recovery. During the month and one-half of Melody's hospitalization there were plateau periods as well in which her condition was neither improving nor worsening and staff were generally uncertain as to what would follow, progress or decline. Even a few days before her death, some of the staff held out hope for her recovery, as Dr. Eason, the plastic surgery resident, felt Melody was demonstrating some minor signs of improvement. The ebb and flow of Melody's career as a patient was marked by the daily laboratory reports on blood cultures, tissue cultures, x-rays, urine tests and so on, studied by her surgeons, consults, and nurses which indicated in many subtle ways the direction she was taking on any given day. As we also saw, the staff searched diligently for visual clues of progress or decline in the daily inspections of burned tissue and grafts. However, in Melody's case, until the final few days of her life, none of the various tests and studies used by the burn unit staff to determine improvement or decline were sufficiently definitive or consistent for staff to say whether she would live or die. In short, there were problems in trajectory.

Melody's case was one of the relatively few examples in the course of this research in which the staff were never entirely certain about the outcome. In most of the work with dying patients, staff knew with some degree of certainty that the patient would die. The central questions in these cases were: how soon the patient would die and what kind of care should be given in the interim. A related problem, and one we will examine more closely later in the chapter, had to do with those occasions when different members of the burn care team disagreed about the probability or likelihood of a patient's death.

The dying patient proved especially difficult for the burn unit staff, in general, as a number of patients were able to survive relatively devastating burn injuries, only to die of massive infection weeks after their admission to the hospital. How well a patient survived his/her first several days on the burn unit was not always an accurate indication of his/her eventual recovery. Melody Lewis' case was a good example of this. National statistics in the United States demonstrate that infection is the leading cause of death from burn injuries and this was the experience in the burn units studied here.

As a result of these experiences, nurses and surgeons attempted to construct dying trajectories: expectations about how and when certain patients would die, as a way of organizing their work, coming to terms and preparing families. Just as there was recovery work on burn patients, so was there death work.

In reducing some of the uncertainty in burn care, staff wanted to gauge with a degree of accuracy when patients would die. This was also a way of organizing and giving meaning to the work that would be performed on patients. Dying trajectories then were staff assessments or predictions about a patient's course in terms of the amount of time a patient would be expected to live. Trajectories were also important for staff in being able to prepare families for what would eventually happen to their loved ones. To the degree that staff had some idea of how and when a particular patient would die, they could begin, in subtle and not so subtle ways, to bring the family to the realization that the patient would not survive. All of this was to prevent families from being shocked and unprepared for death and to assure families that all was being done to help the patient. As in all hospital death and dying, burn unit staff wanted things to go smoothly and routinely and with the minimum of family misunderstandings and misgivings. Later in this chapter, we shall see that these dying events were not always easily handled, as families often took hope for recovery, when they saw their spouses or parents survive the first days or weeks of their burn injury. These families would have a difficult time understanding at a later date, the insidious effects of infection and its eventual devastating impact on the patient's chances for survival.

Dying trajectories on the burn units took several shapes and forms. Most of the trajectories involved some degree of uncertainty as to when and how a particular patient would die. These trajectories could be called "certain trajectories" in that virtually all staff agreed that the odds were not in a patient's favor to survive, but there were some disagreements as to just how long the patient might be expected to live. Two other types of trajectories were less common, but need to be examined as they represent opposite ends of the dying continuum. These can be referred to as the "quick" and "lingering" trajectories.

The quick trajectory was represented in the case of twenty-seven year old Albert Worth. Mr. Worth was admitted to the adult burn unit at six o'clock in the evening of August twentieth. He had sustained 97 percent full-thickness burns in a self-inflicted injury. According to members of his family, Mr. Worth had a history of suicidal behavior. He was examined on admission that evening by Joel Horling, the senior plastic surgery resident and Adam Friedman, the general surgery resident. Horling left for home around eight that evening, but Friedman was on duty the entire night.

The following morning at 7:40 A.M. I was accompanying Joel and Adam as they made rounds in the burn unit. Walking past Mr. Worth's room, Joel noticed it was clean and empty. Joel sipped from his coffee cup and without stopping their walked down the hall, he asked Adam, "When did he die?" Adam replied, "About two hours after you left. His kidneys just shut down. I talked to the family and they took it reasonably well. I guess they saw it coming." Joel nodded, "That's strange. I thought he would at least make it through the night. Shows you what I know."

Quick trajectories occurred most frequently for patients brought to the adult unit literally charred or with massive full-thickness burns and severe pulmonary injuries. Such patients rarely survived more than a few hours or a day or two at most. Commonly these patients were unconscious throughout their ordeal, although I did observe one patient say a few last words to the priest. In the quick trajectories, families were usually prepared immediately and with finality by the surgeons. Families were told they could hold no hope for the victim's survival, but they were free to be with the patient as much as they wanted during the final hours. Surgeons also made families aware that the patient was unconscious and free from pain and agony, which was a concern expressed by most families. These quick trajectories occurred rarely on the children's unit as most children who were massively burned usually died at the scene of the accident or enroute to the hospital.

The lingering trajectory described those patients whom staff expected to die with absolute certainty, but who held on to life for days and even weeks. These patients were often, but, not always, comatose and received basic comfort care rather than heroic measures to keep them alive. Lingering trajectories were actually composed of two types of dying careers. One career line consisted of patients admitted to the burn unit near death, and the staff were prepared for a certain-death trajectory. However, the patient proceeded to linger at the brink of death for several days or weeks. The other lingering career consisted of patients who were admitted with massive burns, but who actually survived the emergence and fluid resuscitation phases only to go into a lingering death trajectory after several weeks on the burn unit.

Such was the case of Gordi Spears, a thirty-three year old male burned in a private plane crash. Gordie was burned over 95 percent of his body but was able to walk from the crash site to summon help. Maggie Renfrow, who was his nurse during much of his hospital stay recalled his death for me in an interview. "Gordie died of sepsis after he spent weeks as a patient up here. No one knows how he survived the crash, but they got him stabilized in the emergency room and we admitted him the night he was burned. For the first few days he even walked around a little on the unit." I asked Maggie, "Were they ever able to get some of his burns grafted?" Maggie nodded, "Yes, but there was hardly any spot to get donors from. They took skin from the top of his head and the bottoms of his feet. Then he got infected and he died a horrible, horrible death." I wanted to know whether his family was with him. Maggie replied, "Oh yes, he had a great and supportive family. They were deeply religious. But Gordie lingered for weeks. No one knew how he was staying alive, but he just wouldn't die! His wife was so strong, Jim. She would stand by the edge of his bed and say to him, 'Gordie, it will soon be over and you'll be with God.' We nurses would be bawling! Tears would be running down our cheeks as we tried to do our charting. The nurses on this unit really identified with that family. We would come in on our days off and sit with Gordie's family. But we thought he never would die. It was just awful."

The lingering trajectory had the most potential for ward upset, as families and staff alike often found the experience emotionally trying, and in the case of young patients such as Gordie Spears, difficult to come to terms with. When families and staff were in agreement, however, as to the type of trajectory the patient was on, it did make matters easier. Some families were reluctant though to accept the staff's definition that a patient was certain to die, and they often developed antagonistic attitudes toward the staff, occasionally refusing to go along with staff recommended procedures for the care of the dying. This particular issue merits closer examination.

Most of the patients who died in the adult burn unit during this study were elderly persons. These individuals often were burned in fire-related household accidents, and while they were not always massively burned, the injury was a terrific assault on their physical system. There is a formula used in estimating a burn victim's chances for survival that fixes the probability of death in terms of a patients's age plus their percent of body surface area burned. For example, if a sixty year old person was burned on 40 percent of her/his body the probability of death would be 100 percent. Burn unit staffs typically take many other factors into the formula, such as a patient's general state of health, whether or not a pulmonary injury was sustained in addition to the burn, the amount of full-thickness burn and so on. Full-thickness burns normally require surgical grafts, and thus would subject an older patient to the rigors of surgery. An inhalation injury would often force a delay in the surgeon's opportunity to surgically debride the burn wounds and this, in turn, could increase the likelihood of a patient developing an infection in the wound tissue. And finally, patients with chronic medical problems or degenerative diseases, such as heart or kidney disease, or cancer would have less physical recources to draw upon in fighting the effects of the burn trauma.

As a result of these considerations, burn unit staff rarely applied the formula of age plus surface burned at face value or in its literal sense. The formula was used primarily as a general guide in assessing death probabilities and in constructing trajectories. However, with elderly patients, a severe burn almost always alerted staff to the firm possibility of death and it would certainly be part of their considerations in dealing with the family. Moreover, as soon as it became clear to staff, in terms of laboratory reports, x-rays, and other visual signs about a patient's condition, that a patient was beginning to physically decline, the dying trajectory would soon be constructed. Staff would initiate predictions as to when and how a patient might die as a way of structuring their work.

Part of the trajectory had to do with decisions to designate a dying patient as a candidate for cardiac resuscitation in the event of cardiac or respiratory arrest. To "code" a patient meant that he/she would receive complete resuscitation measures, e.g., electro-shock, cardiac stimulant drugs, etc. A full-code was reserved for those patients whom staff thought had a favorable chance to recover from their burn wounds.

Conversely a "no-code" represented a decision that no resuscitation measures would be employed and that a patient would receive comfort care only. In the event of cardiac arrest the patient would be allowed to die quietly and life-saving measures would be withheld. On these occasions the patient's family was permitted and encouraged to be at the bedside during the last minutes.

Children and young and middle-aged adults were almost always coded, unless, as in the case of someone like Albert Worth, a patient was burned beyond any reasonable hope for survival. These patients were literally charred and their organ systems almost completely destroyed as a result of their injury. Unless the family insisted upon it, such patients were not coded regardless of their age.

During the period of this study, most of the resuscitation problems emerged in the care of elderly burn victims. Confusion in trajectories were inherent in the interdisciplinary burn team approach and there were frequent disagreements among surgeons and nurses about the survival chances of elderly patients. The younger surgery residents tended to be relatively more optimistic about the recovery of patients, especially when those patients lived through the Emergent Phase of recovery and had their burn injury somewhat stabilized. Let's look at the case of Lucy Mathews as an illustration of this point.

Lucy Mathews was admitted to the adult burn unit on a weekend afternoon. Her clothing had caught fire as she was burning trash in the back yard. Neighbors hearing her screams quickly called the fire department. Lucy was eighty years old, lived alone and enjoyed being independent.

Upon her admission to the burn unit, it was determined that she sustained a 45 percent total body surface area burn. Much of this was deep full-thickness burn injury. To further complicate her condition, Lucy was burned deepest along her neck and chest and as that burned skin tightened it threatened to cut off her breath and she was in danger of choking. Joel Horling, the surgery resident almost immediately performed an escharotomy on her neck and chest, making a long slit in the skin from just under her chin to the navel to open the burned skin and to relieve the pressure.

Despite her advanced age and extent of her burns, Lucy lived through the first week of her admission and the Emergent Phase. She was successfully fluid resuscitated and was semi-conscious after the first week. However, she was designated by the staff as a "no-code," because of her age and percent of full-thickness burn.

During nursing report one morning on Lucy's ninth day post burn, Vickie, who had been Lucy's nurse that evening, told Maureen, who was coming on day shift duty, "Poor Lucy is having an awful time. She just flails around so much in bed." Maureen questioned her, "What are we doing for her?" Vickie answered, "Just give her morphine and keep her comfortable." Maureen nodded, "So she's a no-code? Is her family accepting that?" Sheri, another nurse on duty that day responded, "Oh, I think so. You know Lucy was put on a respirator the other day and they didn't even want that. So I think they agree with the no-code." Vickie added, "Well, her family is all right, but they don't visit Lucy very much. In fact, poor thing gets hardly any visitors." Sheri explained, "They just don't want to see their grandmother like that. I think they want to remember her like she was. That escharotomy looks so gross! Even I have a hard time looking at it."

A few days following, and over a week-end, Adam Friedman, the general surgery resident, felt that Lucy was showing signs of improvement and he wanted to give her some more help. Dr Williams, the Medical Director of the adult unit was out of town for the week-end, so Friedman called Dr. Coyner, the Surgery Chief of the children's unit. Coyner asked Friedman, "How old is she?" Friedman answered, "She's over eighty and has a big burn, but I think she's viable. We've got her fluid resuscitated and everything." Coyner quesioned him further, "Well, what did you have in mind?" Friedman replied, "I would like to start her on Hyper-Al and see if we can't get her to heal." Coyner agreed, "Well, if you feel she's got a chance, I guess you can go ahead." Dr. Friedman thus proceeded to write orders to start Lucy on a high protein liquid that would be ad-

ministered intravenously. This procedure, IV feedings of high protein liquids was usually ordered for patients who were recovering
normally but needed significant nutrient support to promote healing
of their burn wounds.

On Monday morning Grand Rounds, Dr. Williams lead the
team in Lucy's room and quickly spotted the feeding bottle attached
to the IV pole. He turned to Joel and Adam Friedman with a
puzzled look and asked, "Who ordered this?" Joel remained silent
while Adam stepped forward, "I called Coyner on Saturday and he
said to go ahead with it. I just felt she had a chance." Dr. Williams
motioned for Joel and Adam to join him out in the hall. Outside Lucy's room Williams said to Friedman in an even voice, "Well, I sure
don't go for this. Here she is a no-code and you're putting her on
Hyper-Al feedings. It just doesn't make any sense in her case,
Adam. She's eighty years old and she's got a 45 percent burn!" Adam
looked down at the floor and then at Dr. Williams, "I just thought it
was worth a try. Shall we discontinue it?" Dr. Williams, shook his
head, "No, we can't discontinue once we've started. Just cut it down
about a third of what you are giving her."

Later that morning, Friedman drew Maureen aside and said to
her in a quiet and tired voice, "Maureen, start decreasing Lucy's
feeding every few hours." Maureen looked at him and nodded,
"O.K. Adam. Listen, don't feel so bad. You can't save everybody.
You know that." Adam walked away and said over his shoulder, "I
guess not."

That afternoon during nursing report, Maureen told the assembled nurses, "I just feel so bad for Lucy and also for Dr. Friedman; he wants to try so hard." Sheri agreed, "Yeah, Adam got all
excited when they fluid resuscitated her. He felt they had everything
down pat now." Maureen sighed, "Well, the fluid resuscitation is
usually our most successful part. We usually get good results stabilizing the burn trauma. But it's later that the bugs get them."

Several important themes worth mentioning emerge out of the
above case. The surgery residents often were very optimistic about
the survival chances of patients, even the elderly. Possibly due to
their training or personalities as surgeons, they took an activist
orientation toward patient care and wanted to do all they could to
keep patients alive. The residents tended to place considerable

significance on a patient's ability to live through the Emergent Phase or the first few days of their hospital admission. In effect, residents were more likely to feel that if a person survived the tremendous physical shock of the burn injury itself, it improved their chances for recovery. Senior physicians and the more experienced nurses on the burn unit, however, placed less faith and importance on early survival. Their trajectory of expectations was more complex and complicated as they attached greater significance to the effects of sepsis in the Acute Phase. This issue was referred to by Maureen when she was discussing Lucy's condition in nursing report, "The bugs get them." And indeed that is what eventually happened with Lucy Mathews who died in her third week of hospitalization. The effects of infection were most likely to appear several weeks into a patient's admission. Of course, not all patients who become septic died as a result, as we will see in the next chapter, but, a number of patients developed sepsis and succumbed weeks after their initial burn injury.

Nurses and senior surgeons nearly always took this factor into account as they constructed their trajectories. Early optimism was usually tempered with profound respect for the impact of sepsis in the latter recovery stages. This fact presented nurses with awkward moments in their interactions with patients' families. For even as nurses maintained their private suspicions that a patient was likely to die from infection, they had to give nursing care as if the patient was expected to recover. Thus there was a conflict here, in addition to the trajectory conflict between residents and nurses. Here the conflict was more subtle and private, between the nurses' own suspicions that a particular patient would not live, and their public duties as nurses to give competent care as if the patient might. This was appearance care of patients; nursing care given to patients whom nurses held little chance to survive, but whose families expected everything to be done. There is no implication here, however, that the nursing care given was not enthusiastic, thorough, and competent. It was not a case of nurses merely going through the motions. But appearance care meant that as nurses carried out their daily routines on patients, families began to assume that the patient would recover, though nurses might have the patient on a certain-death trajectory.

Appearance care and the sepsis problem lead to the dilemma of what to tell families about the survival chances of patients. As we saw earlier in the situation of a quick death trajectory, the staff expected the patient to die within hours, and they communicated this expectation to families with firmness and finality. There were no cases during my research in which the staff were fooled in their assessments; those patients whom staff expected to die within twenty-four hours did so. In the case of the lingering trajectory, the situation was a bit more complicated and worrisome for staff since it became almost impossible for anyone to tell the family when a patient would die. However, in the lingering trajectory, everyone expected the patient to die, family and staff alike, so that at the very least, there was agreement as to certainty of outcome.

The middle of the dying continuum presented staff with the most nettling problems since there was not always agreement among staff as to certainty of death nor time that it might occur. This inability to agree on trajectory lead to further dilemmas in deciding whether to designate a patient for full-code resuscitation as well as how to prepare families. In everyday experience both problems were interrelated, for to designate a patient as a no-code meant that the staff held no hope for the patient's survival. We will see, later in this chapter, that getting families to agree to a no-code designation, was, in effect, persuading them to accept the fact that the patient would indeed die. It was a means of inducing trajectory agreement.

Conflict in dying trajectories then had to do with what to tell patients' families. Should the staff encourage families to be optimistic about recovery chances or to be realistic and recognize and accept the certain-death trajectories? This conflict was made all the more acute when there were disagreements among the burn team members themselves as to a patient's probable death. Whatever clashes took place were usually between residents' optimism and nurses' realism, as the next case makes evident.

Byron Glenns was eighty-one years old, and severely burned when a water heater exploded in his home. He was admitted to the adult burn unit with 30 percent full-thickness burns to his face, neck, arms and chest. Byron was only semi-conscious at first, and because he was unable to breath sufficiently on his own, he was placed on a respirator. In addition, the surgery residents, Joel Horling and Martin Shapiro, started three intravenous lines, two arterial lines, a urine catheter, and inserted a naso-gastric tube into his stomach. Due to these critical measures and the graveness of his condition, Byron required a nurse present in his room on a twenty-four hour basis. During Grand Rounds the day after Byron was admitted, Joel Horling pointed to Byron's room and told the assembled team, "That guy is going to be lucky to make it through the afternoon." As it turned out, Byron lived for nearly three more weeks, and Horling's certain-death trajectory became the source of some conflicts and tensions.

Byron was alive a week later, though a number of the staff continued to maintain the certain-death trajectory. Dr. Williams, the Medical Director, had just finished examining Byron during Grand Rounds and had walked outside the room to the hall of the burn unit. As the rest of the burn team gathered around him, he lowered his protective mask and said to no one in particular, "Has anyone told his (Byron's) wife that he's going to die?" Betty, the unit social worker, edged her way to the front of the group and answered, "I think she is aware of it. We have talked to her and other members of the family. We talked her into staying at the Family Dorm, so she can be close by. They live about one hundred miles from here." Virginia, one of the other nurses, said to Betty, "I hope he doesn't hang on for several weeks. That would be so hard on her. You know she's not well and she's about the same age as Byron is. With all this strain, she is liable to die before he does!" Dr. Williams continued, "Well, let's take him off the respirator for awhile and see how he does on his own." Virginia asked Williams, "Is he a full-code?" Williams replied, "Yes, I guess at this point he is. Betty, what does his family want done for him?" Betty looked at Dr. Williams, "Everything."

Four days later during nursing report, June, Sheri and Glenda were discussing Byron's condition. Sheri informed the group, "Byron's family seems to feel he is doing real well. He has been off the respirator now for four days." June agreed, "Well, Byron's wife and daughter have the impression that Dr. Shapiro (general surgery resident) is going to save Byron's life. To hear them tell it, Shapiro's going to do everything to keep Byron alive." Sheri slowly shook her head, "These people just don't understand burns! Byron's wife thinks he is doing great because his eyes are open and he recognized some people. She and the daughter keep bringing in the grandchildren and saying, 'Byron, do you know who this is?' And he'll nod every now and then. Well, that's a good sign, but it sure is a small one! Have you seen his lab reports? I mean he is growing all kinds of bad things in his blood. And I mean bad. I just told his family that he had a long way to go yet. It will take him a long time to heal."

Within five days of this conversation the nurses began talking about Byron's impending death. His condition had begun to deteriorate and he was once again placed on a respirator as he could no longer breathe on his own. In the nurses' lounge, Virginia remarked to some of the other nurses, "Byron is dying an awful death. It's so bad it has to be this way. He is in pain from his eschar (burned skin) and he has terrible diarrhea. Also, he's developing a very irregular heart rhythm."

I left the nurses' lounge and proceeded down the hall to Byron's room. Glenda was his nurse today and she was busily adjusting one of Byron's intravenous lines. Byron was connected to a respirator which was noisily and mechanically breathing for him. He was barely visible amid all the dressings, sheets, pillows, IV poles and lines, and the various tubes in his nose and mouth, and lead wires to the heart monitor. I asked Glenda quietly at the foot of the bed, "How long do you think he has?" Glenda shook her head, "It could be hours. But it could be days, though I hope not for his sake." I noticed the radio was now on in his room. "Why the radio, Glenda?" Glenda looked at me and smiled, "Oh, the sound of that respirator gets to me after awhile. It drives me nuts. So the radio helps drown it out. Also, since Byron is bed-ridden maybe the radio gives him some contact with the outside world. But I don't know if he can hear it or not."

The following morning was Monday Grand Rounds, marking Byron's third Monday on the unit. The team didn't spend more than a few minutes in Byron's room before everyone filed out into the hall. This was usually a sign that most everyone felt the patient was in the final stage of the death trajectory.

As the team gathered in the hall, Dr. Williams asked Betty, the social worker, "What about Byron's wife now, Betty? What's her condition?" Before Betty could respond, Dr. Shapiro interjected, "She's still alive." Williams grinned at him and said, "I assume that. What I want to know is how she feels about resuscitation. I mean Byron is just about gone." Joel Horling spoke up. "This is a very cooperative family, Don. I've explained to them the various levels of resuscitation and they don't want us beating on his chest or anything like that. If we can do something with drugs, then that's O.K." Joel paused for a moment, "In my mind he's not a no-code. But we told them (family) that even if he gets through this his prognosis is still bad. They want him comfortable. They don't want him to suffer."

Dr. Williams brightened up a little and told Dr. Horling and the group, "Now this is important. That is to let the family know that we can make it so he won't suffer." He looked at Virginia, "Go ahead and use morphine. I would feel free to do that." Virginia nodded, "Well, he's had a lot of pain. His eschar is loosening up and separating and this is painful for him." Williams agreed, "Then let's keep him comfortable. This is an approach that Byron's family can understand. We'll keep him comfortable." Turning to Joel Horling, Williams asked, "Now why are you giving him blood? I thought we weren't going to start anything new." Horling rubbed his cheek and looked at Williams, "Over the week-end he started bleeding from the rectum so we gave him some blood." Williams questioned him, "Do you plan to continue?" Horling shook his head, "No, not after today." Wiliams straightened up and turned, "Fine, now who else have we got down here today?"

On Wednesday following Monday Rounds, Virginia was in the nurses' lounge having lunch with Vickie and two other nurses. Virginia was disturbed about a conversation she had the day before with Dr. Shapiro, the general surgery resident, "I just know that Byron's not going to make it, but Shapiro thinks he's going to save him. Do you know that yesterday Shapiro told Byron's family that Byron was doing better. What's the matter with him? I'll tell you what it is. Shapiro can't accept death." Vickie added, "Horling doesn't agree with Shapiro, does he?" Virginia was emphatic, "Why no! He told Shapiro when Byron came in that he wasn't going to make it. Now Shapiro is telling everyone, 'If it was my grandfather, I would want everything done for him.' He's also badrapping Dr. Williams because he won't order any more blood for Byron. Well, I don't blame Williams." Vickie sympathized with Virginia, "This morning the medical student, Cathy, said the burn unit was giving up on Byron." Virginia was getting more upset, "That's not true and she knows it. We give him the best care even if he is a no-code. I told Shapiro yesterday that Byron's family doesn't want him to suffer. And Shapiro said he didn't think Byron was suffering that much. Well, my God, Shapiro's not there when we do Byron's dressing changes. He would change his tune if he could see that. And I'm concerned about Byron's wife. The poor thing is worried sick and she's not very healthy."

Friday morning of that same week, Byron's wife was in the family waiting room as I was going into the burn unit. I sat with her for a few minutes as I had done several times before, and asked her about Byron. She answered, "Oh, I feel he is just a little better today. You know I never give up. We're farmers, Byron and I. We farmed all our life it seems. Just don't know why this had to happen to him. But I pray for him every day and know that God will answer my prayers. You just can't quit praying." Byron's condition worsened over the week-end and he died early Sunday morning, nearly three weeks after he was admitted.

The example of Byron Glenns gives us insight into the problems of dying trajectories in the burn unit. When Byron was admitted, his age, eighty-one years, plus his 30 percent body surface burn, affixed his probability of dying at over 100 percent. The fact that he required a respirator initially was not lost on Dr. Horling who, on Byron's second day of admission told the burn team that Byron wasn't likely to live through the day.

Virtually everyone agreed with this preliminary trajectory, but were forced to modify when Byron improved sufficiently to be taken off the respirator. Subsequently, he actually breathed on his own for several days. This slight sign of progress was enough to set off two chain of events that produced conflicts for the nursing staff and Dr. Williams, the Medical Director. One, Byron's improvement provided the impetus for Shapiro, the young surgery resident, to change his trajectory from certain-death to a prognosis that left some hope for recovery. Second, the temporary improvement, was interpreted by Byron's wife and family as an indication that he might eventually pull through. It was at this point that the grandchildren were brought in to visit and Byron responded with slight nods of his head. Moreover, the decision was made now, and Dr. Horling agreed, that Byron should be coded in the event of cardiac failure.

This was in harmony with the family's wishes that everything be done.

However, none of the nursing staff nor Dr. Williams actually abandoned their certain-death trajectory, though they might have felt uneasy about it. While Byron's death was not imminent during this second week, it was going to come eventually because all his laboratory reports indicated that he was septic. At this point, the nursing staff did not rule out for Byron's family the possibility of his recovery, but continually reminded them that Byron was indeed very sick and faced a long road ahead. While the nursing staff had Byron on a certain-death trajectory, they nursed him continually as if he were a viable patient, which further reinforced the family's hopes that there was a remote possibility he would live. Nevertheless, the nurses pressed Byron's family to be realistic about the likelihood that he could die.

The end stage of the trajectory came during Byron's third week post-burn, when he was placed on the respirator once again because of his deteriorating physical status. Now Dr. Williams was all the more convinced that his certain-death trajectory was indeed the correct one, and he began to suggest comfort care (e.g. morphine) for Byron during Grand Rounds. His feelings were totally compatible with the nursing staff, particularly with Virginia, who wanted to prevent Byron from having an agonizing death and increasing the stress on his wife. The conflict surfaced, however, when Dr. Shapiro refused to accept the certain-death trajectory and began to hold out hope for the family, by telling them that he would do all he could to save Byron's life. Thus Byron's wife and daughter, much to the dismay of the nurses, put their faith in Dr. Shapiro, although they did agree that if Byron went into cardiac failure, he should not receive heroic medical resuscitation.

Shapiro's attitude proved very difficult for the nurses, who for nearly three weeks had tried to gently and subtly prepare Byron's family for his eventual death. While the nurses were gradually persuading the family to accept a certain-death trajectory, Shapiro at the same time, was taking a stance with the family as one who would save the day. This produced conflicting messages for the family who respected and trusted the nurses, but who were looking also for any thread of hope they could grasp. Partially as a result of this conflict among staff, Byron's wife held out hope to the very end and even two days before he died, thought she detected slight improvement. From the point of view of the burn care team, this inability to reach a common trajectory and front with Byron's family placed a severe strain on the sense of team work between the nurses and the surgical resident.

While thus far in this chapter we have looked at trajectory conflicts among staff and the implications of these conflicts for patient care and family interactions, there were an equal number of occasions when the burn care team agreed fairly closely on the trajectory. When the staffs achieved consensus on a certain-death trajectory, the problem arose often in getting a patient's family to accept the trajectory. The issue of resuscitation codes became significant here and a point of contention between the family and the burn care team. Often families wanted everything possible done to save the life of their loved one, and this included full resuscitation if that became necesary. Burn unit staff, however, in establishing a certain-death trajectory wanted to avoid having to resuscitate patients whom they felt had no chance to survive. When families insisted on full-code resuscitation there was little the burn team could do other than comply with the families' wishes. If, on the other hand, the family was ambivalent about their feelings, which many of them were, the staff would encourage the family to adopt a no-code designation. Such persuasive efforts were most frequent when the patient in question was elderly and the extent of burn was significant. It will be instructive for us to look at the case history of Herb Taylor to better understand some of the dynamics of this issue.

Herb Taylor had been trapped in a house-fire and before being rescued, he suffered 45 percent full-thickness burns to his upper body. Herb was eighty-six years old, enjoyed reasonably good health and had a very large family. He was brought to the burn unit in the evening and after examining his injuries, none of the burn team held any hopes for his recovery. In fact, one of the nurses on duty that evening remarked to Herb's granddaughter, "If it was my grandfather, I would just let him go."

This comment proved quite upsetting to the young woman and the next morning she requested a meeting with the administrative coordinator of the burn unit. The granddaughter explained her concerns, "Last night one of the nurses told me that if Herb was a member of her family, she would just let him go. Well, he's not a member of her family. He is our grandfather and we are concerned about him. If the nurses think he is gong to die, I hope they don't do something to hurry it along!" The burn unit coordinator reassured her, "Oh, you don't need to worry about that. The nurses here will give him the best care possible. As of right now he is a full-code. Do you know what that means?" Herb's granddaughter hesistated, "I guess not exactly." The coordinator went on to explain, "Well, it means that if Herbs' heart stops or anything like that, the doctors will do everything to revive him." The young woman looked somewhat relieved, "That makes me feel better about things." "Good, and remember if there is any change in the code policy, it will only be after the doctors discuss it with you and the rest of the family."

The next day, all the nurses that I talked to expected Herb to die. They even felt that Herb himself wanted to die. Glenda was telling the other nurses in the lounge, "I think poor old Herb wants to die. Yesterday when anesthesia was here to intubate him (connect to a respirator) he kept saying to just leave him alone. Gwenn added, "He just wants someone to hold his hand. He held mine this morning and just wouldn't let go. He probably doesn't want to die alone in a hospital. It's so sad." Vickie commented, "He knows he is not going to make it. Maybe we should get a volunteer to sit in his room and hold his hand." Glenda smiled at her, "Now that wouldn't be a bad idea."

Herb Taylor, although showing no signs of improvement, was alive ten days later. He was now on a life-support system as he could no longer breathe without the aid of a respirator. Dr. Williams had looked in on Herb early that morning and as he was walking up the hall he spotted Adam Friedman, the general surgery resident. "Adam, does Herb's family know his condition?" Adam nodded, "Yes, I think they do. They have been very accommodating to our recommendations so far." Williams was firm, "I think you need to make sure they know there is no hope for Herb. With his age and a 45 percent burn, well, you know his chances." Adam agreed to talk more to Herb's family. A few minutes later I asked Adam if this meant that Herb wouldn't be coded. Adam answered, "Yes, he won't be coded now. If he goes into cardiac arrest we won't resuscitate him. I'm glad I don't have to make those decisions. That's what the Medical Director's paid to do. So Herb won't be coded. This is what I'll suggest to the family and I feel they'll go along with it. They want what's best for him."

That same day, toward the middle of the afternoon, Herb died. He was not resuscitated. During nursing report the following morning, several of the nurses were eager to learn about what had happened with Herb since they were not on duty when he died. Sheri asked Glenda, "Was his family there? They were so supportive of him." Glenda replied, "Yes, they were there but, just barely. Herb started going down-hill around three o'clock. His blood pressure kept going down and I knew he was going out. I went to the waiting room to get the family and they were gone! But they got back in time to spend thelast few minues with him." Maureen looked at Glenda, "How did they take it?" Glenda answered, "His wife was there and she told me that she felt all along that Herb wasn't going to make it."

Herb Taylor's case gives us an example of trajectory agreement among staff. Virtually everyone working in the burn unit felt that Herb would die and he surprised everyone too by living as long as he did. Though staff never altered their certain-death trajectory, they did change their code designation on Herb, although not until nearly the very end of his life. Initally, as we saw, Herb was a full-code and the surgeons and nurses wre careful to make the family aware of this in light of the nurses' comments made to them on Herb's first day of admission. While he lived for twelve days on the unit his condition never improved enough for staff to change their trajectory. During the final days, Dr. Williams, the Medical Director, realized that Herb would not survive and Williams was then faced with getting the family to agree to change Herb from a full-code to a no-code. He was pleased then to learn from Adam Friedman that this was an "accommodating family" and would go along with Williams' suggestion, made to them by way of Dr. Friedman, that Herb not be resuscitated. Thus, conflict here was minimal as the family was made to realize and accept the gravity of Herb's condition. Moreover, as Glenda learned moments after Herb's death, his wife had not expected him to survive either and this probably gave additional support to the family's acceptance of the no-code.

Agreements between burn unit staff and families about resusciatation policies were not then the result of fully informed negotiations. Families were apprised about the conditions of patients but, since death and recovery signs were technical and subtle, families had to rely on the staff's interpretations of how well patients were doing or how near to death they were. Many families had difficulty making reasoned judgments about such matters and could only react to the loyalties, obligations, and emotions they were feeling at a particular time. If they insisted that their loved one be resuscitated no matter what the condition or prognosis, they always got their way, regardless of how reluctant the staff might have been. There were such occasions though they were rare. By and large, decisions about resuscitation codes were defined in medical terms and flowed from the top down; that is, from the Medical Director through the surgery residents to the family. As Herb Taylor's case illustrated, the Medical Director assessed the probabilities of survival and guided the efforts of the surgery residents toward an appropriate resuscitation decision. While the Medical Director talked to families directly on a number of occasions, it was usually left for the residents to interpret for families what, in the judgment of medical authority, was best for a particular patient. Thus families were nudged into embracing the certain-death trajectories and the ultimate no-resuscitation codes as they acceded to the wisdom and experience of higher medical authority.

Chapter Seven

RECOVERY TRAJECTORIES

WHILE burning early Fall leaves in the back yard of his home, Milt Carlin accidently ignited his work clothes and before help could arrive, he was burned over 60 percent of his body. Milt's burns were nearly all partial-thickness, but he was fortunate in that he did not sustain an inhalation injury. Brought to the Regional Burn Center on September seventh, the admitting staff learned then that Milt was sixty-two years old and had been employed as an industrial plumber for some thirty years. Milt was of medium physical build, wore glasses and was balding.

His first week on the burn was uneventful as he responded to treatment rather well. Each day he was taken to the tank room for hydrotherapy and dressing changes. Though his physical condition was stable and encouraging, emotionally, Milt felt depressed, withdrawn and somewhat frightened during his first few days as a patient. He told some of the staff, on the day he was admitted, that he was worried about dying. Two days later, however, in the middle of painful hydrotherapy session, he told Dr. Williams that indeed he wanted to die. Dr. Williams looked down into the tub at him and said good-naturedly, "Well, we've got a big club right outside the door." Later that day, Dr. Williams told some members of the nursing staff that he fully expected Milt to recover.

A week after Milt's admission to the burn unit, and as his condition continued to stabilize his spirits and outlook were improving. Gwenn, one of the nurses working with him that morning told me, "Milt is quite talkative now. He was really discouraged last week, so

196

I'm pleased to see him talking to us. He just needs someone to get him talking, that's all."

On the morning of his seventh day in the hospital, I was present in the tank room watching Myra, a physical therapist, giving Milt some exercises in the hydrotheapy tank. Myra and Gwenn engaged Milt in a continuous stream of conversation while they worked with him as he lay in the water. Whenever their discussion lagged, they would think up new questions to put to him. When they learned that he was unmarried but had a woman friend, they wanted to know all about her. At one point, Myra was exercising Milt's burned arms over his head, and she told him, "You need to stretch those arms up high Milt, so when you take Jane (Milt's friend) dancing you can twirl her on the dance floor!" Milt responded weakly, "Oh, I don't feel much like dancing now." Myra persisted, "Well, you play golf don't you? This will help you with your golf swing."

After a break in their conversation, I introduced myself to Milt while he was still in the tank. He had earlier mistaken me for one of the surgeons. Milt asked me a number of questions about my background and then remarked, "Jim, I'm in an awful lot of pain. This is about the worst thing that has ever happened to me and I was in the War!"

Milt's physical status remained stable and unchanging for twelve days post-admission, until the nineteenth of September when it appeared to the burn unit staff that he was having a setback. Various laboratory studies and Milt's physical appearance gave the staff cause for alarm. During Grand Rounds, Dr. Williams, Dr. Horling, and Dr. Friedman huddled together discussing Milt's deteriorating physical condition. They had just spent several minutes in his room carefully examining his burn wounds and studying some disturbing, yet puzzling laboratory findings. Friedman shared his opinion with Dr. Williams, "I would say that he's septic." Williams disagreed shaking his head slightly, "All his quantitatives (tissue cultures) are negative. If he were septic they would have to be positive, Adam." The interchange of opinions continued for several more minutes as the three surgeons reviewed Milt's complicated medical condition. Finally, Dr. Williams suggested to the two residents that Milt's setback was due, in part, to a burn induced diabetes. Since either of the residents seemed familiar with that type of condition, Williams directed them to get Milt's diabetic problem straightened out. "If we can get that cleared up, then we can see what we're working with here." Myra questioned Dr. Williams, "Should we continue to take him for hydrotherapy?" Dr. Williams answered her, "No, not for now. We have to get this other business under control and we don't want to run the risk of infection. Let's keep him in bed." Williams then turned to Betty, the unit social worker, "Betty, does Milt's family have any idea how sick he really is?" Betty paused for a moment, "Well, I'm not for sure. I think they all went home for a few days. Maybe we should call them and tell them to come back."

The next day many of the staff I talked to felt that Milt had definitely taken a turn for the worse. Dr. Horling was resting and drinking black coffee in the nurses' lounge, when Vera, one of the nurses on duty, sat down next to him and asked, "Tell me, Joel, is Milt Carlin going to die?" Horling slowly turned to her and said with a sigh, "He does look a lot worse, doesn't he?" Vera nodded, "Why he looks worse now than when he came in."

When Horling finished his coffee, he stood up and stretched, and then asked me, "You want to walk down to surgery with me?" As we proceeded down the two flights of stairs to the surgery floor, Horling described Milt for me, "Well, he's sixty-two years old and he's burned nearly 60 percent. Add that together and that's not a good chance of making it. I guess anything could happen."

I returned to the burn unit later that afternoon and entered Milt's room. Adam Friedman had just finished putting an arterial line in Milt's right ankle and he was methodically taping it in place. Friedman told me some things about burn induced diabetes and ended the talk by saying, "To be honest, yesterday when Williams mentioned it, that was news to me. But last night I got caught up pretty fast by reading what the journals had to say. I hate getting put on the spot like that. But we will get this under control, or at least I hope we will."

Milt was laying very still in bed, his face was quite pale and he was talking incoherently. Streams of words were coming out of his mouth but they didn't form sentences or have any relation to what was going on in his room. Milt had several long lead wires attached to his chest which were connected to a large heart monitor console mounted above and to the right of his bed. In addition to the arterial line in his ankle, Milt had intravenous lines in each arm and a naso-gastric tube inserted through his nose. While I was looking at Milt, the burn unit coordinator entered the room and told Dr. Friedman that she had notified Milt's family that his condition had worsened. They had agreed to return to the hospital at once.

For the next three days Milt remained confined to bed, but his condition had stabilized somewhat. While the various daily laboratory studies continued to show cause for concern, the surgery residents felt that Milt was holding his own.

On September twenty-first, I watched Gwenn give Milt his morning dressing change and she worked alone at the task which normally required two nurses. The burn unit that week had several critical patients and no other nurse could free up enough time to help Gwenn at that particular moment. The dressing change took two hours and Milt was alert and conscious, though very weak and in considerable pain. Gwenn talked quietly to him talking about his hobbies such as fishing and golf. She finished Milt's dressings shortly before visiting hours were to begin, and although Milt looked and acted tired, Gwenn told him that she wanted to make him look"presentable" for his visitors. Using scissors, Gwenn cut away parts of Milt's gauze dressings that were blood stained, combed his hair, and cleaned up his eye glasses.

Vera, another nurse, entered the room as Gwenn was doing this. "Gwenn, do you need some help? I've got a few minutes now." Gwenn smiled at her, "No, I'm just about finished with Milt. We're sprucing him up for his family, aren't we, Milt?" Vera walked to the side of the bed and began to gently rub and pat his forehad. She told him, "Milt, your face is really starting to look nice now. You're coming along real fine." Vera begain to slowly and almost absent-mindedly remove small bits of dead burned tissue from Milt's face as he lay there nearly asleep. Occasionally he would say something, but most of the conversation was between Vera and Gwenn. Vera remarked,"I've been picking at these little crusties on Milt's face. They come off so easily. And look how nice his face is now!"

Later that afternoon I returned to Milt's room and he was arguing with Gwenn about having to be in his abductor cushions. This type of splint extended on opposite sides of the bed and he was required to have his arms extended in them for several hours each day.

The purpose was to prevent contractures from forming on his burned arms. As I walked into the room, I told him, "Milt, you're looking pretty good this afternoon." He looked up at me and snapped, "Who the Hell cares if you look good if you feel lousy?" I replied, "You don't feel any better, Milt?" He was short with me, "No, I don't feel any better. But I would like to get some rest if people would leave me alone." Gwenn was giving Milt a shave and she stopped long enough to say, "Now cut it out, Milt. These things are necessary. You need a shave and you're going to get one." After Gwenn finished with the razor, she cleaned his dentures, and once again carefully combed his hair and then searched for some after-shave lotion. Gwenn told him, "We're going to get you all cleaned up and smelling pretty. How about that?" Milt replied firmly, "I really don't care. I would prefer some peace and quiet."

The following morning Milt didn't feel very well and his pain seemed to be worse. He was very withdrawn and moody, and as I watched Vera change his dressings, he told her in a weak voice to come near so he could whisper in her ear. Vera put her face down close to his, "What is it, Milt?" Milt said quietly, "There is a fear now that I haven't told the doctors about." Vera asked, "Well, what is it?" Milt answered, "I just don't know if I'm going to get well or not. Vera, I don't want to die. I don't want to die!" Vera straightened up for a few moments without saying anything, then she looked at him again, "Oh, Milt." He continued, "I'm not afraid to die. That's not it. I can talk to God just like I'm talking to you. But I'm not ready to die and I don't want to." Vera patted him on the forehead and she appeared to be at a loss for words. "Milt, you're going to be O.K. Just have some faith and everything will turn out all right." Vera quickly moved to the doorway and asked Gwenn for some help with Milt. As the two nurses were changing his bed, he told Gwenn in a whimpering voice, "Gwenn, I don't think I'm going to make it." Gwenn smiled at him, "Milt, an ornery guy like you? Of course you'll make it. Don't worry so much."

Thoughout the rest of the day, Milt experienced periods of disorientation and delirium. Whenever any of the staff entered his room they would attempt to orient him by asking questions that forced him to respond. Sandi, the occupational therapist, visited that afternoon and asked him, "Milt, do you remember who I am?"

Milt responded weakly, "Yes, you're Sandi, who gives me those mean exercises and makes my bones hurt." Sandi smiled at me, "Well, at least Milt, you're more alert than yesterday. You didn't even know who I was!"

Vera and I were talking the following day in the nurses' lounge and I asked her about Milt. Vera appeared concerned, "I don't think he's doing very well. His burns don't look good; they have that filmy gloss to them. But I feel if he could just get over the hump, he'll get better." I brought up the subject of Milt's death talk. Vera shrugged her shoulders. "Oh, it gets to me when he talks about dying like that. But I'm not ready to write him off yet. I still think he's going to make it." Vera paused to sip her coffee, "I know in our training they told us to let the patient talk and get their feelings out in the open. And maybe there are some things they want to get said before they die. But it's just hard for me to talk to them. I don't feel we have the time to sit down and talk with our patients like they need."

Five days after that conversation with Vera, and eighteen days following his admission to the burn unit, Milt's condition began to improve. Vera met me in the hall as I was coming into the burn unit after being away for the week-end, acting quite pleased, "Milt is looking much better now. I'm so glad he made it through the week-end. On Friday I thought he looked terrible; today he seems so improved! He's even acting ornery now and yelling at the nurses. Milt's back to his old self and that's a good sign!"

Gwenn and I talked for awhile after lunch in the nurses' lounge. She said to me, "You should have been with Milt today, Jim. He said he was feeling better and he actually wanted to get out of bed so he could sit up. Can you believe it? He told me that he thinks he is getting better because his pain isn't so bad."

During the entire day Milt's improvement was the central topic of conversation among everyone in the burn unit. Whenever someone passed his room they would invariably peek in and compliment him on how well he was looking. Milt drew praise from every corner. Even Drs. Horlings and Friedman felt satisfied that Milt had turned the corner. Friedman asked Horling in the physician's dictation office, "Milt seems to be coming out of it, and the nurses want to take him to the tank. What do you think?" Horling hesitated, "What about that arterial line in his ankle?" Friedman responded, "I can put it in his wrist. It should be O.K." Horling agreed, "Well, it's O.K. with me, if they think they can manage it."

By the end of the following week Milt was well enough to go to the tank for hydrotherapy every day. I watched his session one morning and when the nurses and therapists were finished we took Milt back to his room in a wheelchair. Vera asked him if he wanted to sit in the wheelchair for awhile and Milt agreed, "Now Jim and I can have a talk for awhile. You're in no hurry to leave are you, Jim?" Milt did most of the talking and told me much about his background. He recounted his days as a plumber and the changes he had witnessed in the plumbing industry. Milt also mentioned the possibility of asking his woman friend to marry him. "She's a wonderful woman, Jim, and she has stuck by me through all this mess. Maybe I'll retire and we'll settle down together."

In the tank room the next morning Milt told Myra and Gwenn, "Jane (Milt's woman friend) told me that my hair needs washing. Can we do that this morning?" Gwenn got excited and reached for the shampoo, "Why of course, Milt! You want to look good for Jane. Sounds like she's getting serious about you, Milt." Milt looked smug, "Oh, she probably is."

For several consecutive days Milt was a celebrity of sorts on the unit, as each day he got stronger and more healthy. Virtually everything he did drew compliments from the staff and even other patients told him continually how well he looked. The biggest moment came on October fifth when Milt walked unassisted from the tank room to his own room, a distance of forty feet. The nurses were clapping and he was promised a soft drink for his efforts. From that moment forward, Milt no longer required nor was he allowed to use the wheelchair.

I asked Joel Horling what had brought about Milt's rapid improvement. Over coffee he explained to me, "I think it was a combination of things that we tried. First we finally got that diabetes straightened out and then Adam Friedman did a real nice job with Milt's metabolism. That really got things going. And he just started to heal and that's why his is feeling so much better." I asked, "Will he need surgery?" Horling shook his head, "I guess not. Dr. Williams looked at him this morning and he doesn't feel Milt will need any grafts. And that's fine with me. With his age and extent of burns it's

O.K. with me if we don't operate."

Several days later, it was decided that Milt was well enough that the staff could think about sending him home. During Grand Rounds on Monday when the entire team was gathered in Milt's room, he looked around the room and said, "I'm supposed to ask Dr. Wood if I can go home." Gwenn corrected him, "Dr. Williams, Milt." Milt looked sheepish, "Oh, I'm sorry, Dr. Williams. Can I go home?" Williams nodded at him, "Yes, mid to end of this week." Milt let out a big sigh and smiled, "I'm so happy to hear that." As Williams was walking into the hall he said over his shoulder, "The pleasure will be ours." Sandi whispered to Williams, "Gee, I hope he didn't hear that."

Toward the end of the week that Milt was to go home, Sheri, Maureen and Glenda were discussing his announcement that he intended to get married upon his release from the hospital. Maureen seemed rather pleased,"Isn't that just great? Milt wants to get married now." Sheri looked concerned, "You don't suppose he thought up these marriage plans when he was out of it, do you?" Glenda disagreed, "Oh, no. He didn't start talking about getting married until he was well."

The day Milt left the burn unit there was a small party for him. Milt personally thanked all the nurses and other staff he could find. Maureen reminded Milt that everyone on the unit expected a wedding invitation. Milt promised that all would be included. On October twenty-third, forty-six days after he was admitted, Milt returned home.

This chapter is concerned with how the burn care team managed the recovery care of their patients. While as we saw in the preceding chapter, not all patients lived, nonetheless, the burn unit staff expected most patients to recover. Those recoveries were, however, slow and arduous, and the progress benchmarks were infrequent and not always clearly defined. The case of Milt Carlin, which introduced this chapter, was fairly typical of the long and complicated recovery sequence that many burn patients went through. On the adult unit, patients remained on the unit an average of twenty-two days during their recovery. Many patients such as Mr. Carlin, stayed much longer, and a number of patients in this study were hospitalized for several months.

As a result of this fact, burn unit staff constructed recovery trajectories for patients, expectations about how and when patients would recover. Just as there were dying trajectories to structure and give meaning to the passage from life to death on the burn unit, so there were trajectories that gave form to the passage from sickness and injury to recovery. These trajectories served to focus the staff's attention on certain events and processes of recovery as a means of organizing work and coming to terms. As patients recovered through time, and as their recoveries were marked by periods of gain, setbacks and reversals, the trajectories made sense and gave structure to what might otherwise seem as vague and almost indefinable periods of recovery. In short, the trajectories served to make recovery work more manageable.

Recovery trajectories were structured around three social phases of burn patient recovery that corresponded roughly with the three stages of physical/medical recovery. These social stages will be referred to as: Initial-Preparatory Stage; the Normalizing Stage; and the Dispositional Stage. During the Initial-Preparatory Stage, staff tried to assess or estimate how well a patient would do on the burn unit. In anticipating contingencies in a patient's recovery, staff tried to prepare themselves for each patient's future needs and problems. The Normalizing Stage, which corresponded with the acute phase of physical recovery, saw the staff concerned primarily with the morale or emotional well-being of patients. And in the Dispositional Stage, staff attempted to determine a patient's readiness to return home. For those patients considered sufficiently rehabilitated, staff began to prepare them to return to a normal life. Having briefly introduced the three recovery stages, I would now like to devote the remainder of this chapter to a detailed examination of each stage.

Initial-Preparatory Stage

The earliest period of the recovery trajectory, the Initial-Preparatory Stage, covered a patient's first several days or earliest weeks on the burn unit. During this time, the burn unit team tried to get an initial idea of a patient's recovery chances. Put differently, the staff sought an understanding of what they would be up against in helping a patient recover as well as a prediction of the kind of contingencies they would have to prepare for.

Sheri, one of the burn unit nurses interviewed, expressed staff concerns in this way, "We try to see how a patient will do even on the day of admission. We look to see if they are completely charred, for example, or if there is a pulmonary injury. If there is a pulmonary injury then we know there will be complications. If it is a young patient, we hope that they'll make it. You know, like when Bobby Williams came in, he had a big burn, but he didn't have a pulmonary injury, so I felt he could survive. And he has so far." I asked her to elaborate, "What other considerations do you feel are important?" Sheri continued, "Well, I feel we look for the survivability of the patient. What do they have going for them and against them? You expect a more difficult time when the larger the burn and more full-thickness involvement. For me, I also look at their reaction to pain. Even on that first day, does it look like they can endure the pain?" Sheri paused for a few moments and then added, "A patient is also going to need a good family and I look for that. Do they have a supportive family and will they encourage the patient to go along with the program. That is important."

As patients were first admitted, their medical history was elicited and diagnostic workup began. In the context of this work, the staff searched for the sort of clues that Sheri mentioned. Also, patients themselves were given an initial idea of how badly they were injured and some of the ordeals that lay in store for them as they recovered.

Ned Rice was admitted on August ninth with 35 percent full and partial thickness burns to his face, neck and chest as a result of an explosion in the foundry where he worked. He was conscious throughout this admission examination. The attending staff quickly placed him on a cart and began to clean and examine his burn wounds. After Virginia, one of the nurses, took several blood samples from his arms, Sandi came into the tank room to measure him for positioning splints. As she was doing this, Dr. Horling entered the tank room and while he was looking at Ned's burns, he asked him. "Have you had any recent illnesses?" Ned responded weakly, "No, I haven't." Horling continued, "Any surgeries in the past or a medical problem we should know about?" Ned shook his head, "No, I can't think of anything. I've been pretty healthy up till now." Horling put his stethoscope to Ned's chest and began to listen intently.

A few minutes after Horling had finished and left the room,

Virginia went to the side of the cart and looked down at Ned, "Ned, your face is going to swell up because you've got some burns there. And your eyes will swell shut for a few days. But you don't need to worry; in a couple of days you will be back to normal. Now in a minute we're going to put you in a tub with warm water to clean you up."

Maureen wanted to test the depth of Ned's burns and to do so she took a needle from a packet on the dressing cart and told him, "Ned, I'm going to push your skin in a few places and I want you to tell me if you feel anything. O.K.?" Ned slowly nodded his head. Maureen gently poked the needle into several areas of the burns on Ned's arms and shoulder. "Can you feel the needle there, Ned?" Ned answered, "No, I don't feel anything." Maureen assured him, "That's O.K. Now I'm going to do a few more places."

A while later Maureen remarked to Virginia, "Ned's got some soot in his mouth and throat. I saw it when I swabbed him for a (throat) culture. I bet he's going to have some inhalation problems. And he's a smoker too."

Among the various patient experiences expected by staff during the Initial-Preparatory Stage were some degree of confusion and disorientation as a response to the shock of the burn trauma and to the rigors of daily critical care. Such confusion and delirium were defined by staff as fairly normal responses within the early phase of recovery.

Bobby Williams' case is a good example. With 90 percent burns to his body, Bobby was hospitalized for over two months. During his first few weeks on the burn unit when he was still in the Emergent Phase of physical recovery, Bobby was frequently disoriented and he talked confused. He told Myra, his physical therapist one morning, "I know why these position splints hurt my arms so much." Myra asked him, "Why is that, Bobby?" "Because my arms were made by Pinto and these splints were made by Toyota. You can see for yourself right here." Myra changed the subject, but later Bobby told her, "I don't need any skin grafting now." Myra corrected him, "Yes, you do, Bobby. Your skin won't heal on its own." Bobby persisted, "I know, but I got my new skin last night while I was sleeping. Who needs grafts? This skin is brand new." Later I asked Myra why Bobby was talking like that. She explained, "Oh, he's just all stressed out. He's bed-ridden and with all the pain he is having he gets all whiney and stressed out. Yesterday he screamed at his fiance because she ordered the wrong breakfast cereal for him. It's just stress."

Dr. Horling had his own theory about Bobby's confusion. "It is nothing to worry about. A lot of patients go through this at this point. There's a kind of psychosis that critical care patients get sometimes. They're shut up in their room for so long. They lose track of things. Patients attached to a ventilator sometimes get that way too."

As an interesting side issue here, patients brought to the burn unit for self-inflicted burn injuries often had their disorientation and delirium explained in terms of their personality and character structure. These patients were thought to be different from other patients who were "normal." Self-inflict persons found that many of their subsequent behaviors and attitudes were defined by staff in terms of their status as a person who tried suicide. Once I asked Gwenn about Carla Wolfe, a woman patient who at a certain point in her recovery appeared disoriented in some of her actions. Gwenn responded, "Oh, Carla? She's out of it. She set herself on fire, you know." This label stuck with Carla throughout her stay and many of her adaptive modes were explained in light of her suicidal tendencies.

In the Initial-Preparatory Stage, staff considered the severity of the burn wound and its relation to the kind of recovery that staff expected a patient to make. During the first several days there was usually much talk and disucssion among staff about a patient's wounds, the extent of body surface covered, amount of full-thickness involvement and whether facial disfigurement was a possibility. Such burn wound talk and concern were means of initially defining a patient's situation and composing the trajectory. Even patients admitted to the unit with multiple trauma injuries, in addition to their burn wound, were defined primarily as burn patients, though staff might concede that, initially, other injuries might be more significant than the burn wound itself.

This was illustrated in the early activities surrounding the care of seventeen year old Lonnie Gorham, severely injured in an automobile crash and explosion. Lonnie was cardiac resuscitated at the scene by paramedics, and subsequently brought to the hospital with multiple trauma injuries including a massive skull fracture and brain concussion. Operated on immediately by a team of neurosurgeons, he was in a deep coma for the next ten days. The adult burn unit admitted Lonnie directly following his eight-hour surgery. Despite the fact that Lonnie was comatose, the nurses and other members of the burn team staff treated Lonnie as a burn patient and started their routine burn care treatment and assessment protocols. Vera, one of the nurses working that afternoon, estimated the extent and depth of his burns through direct examination of the wounds. She found that nearly all of Lonnie's burns were full-thickness and covered much of his right arm from shoulder to hand, parts of his head and the right half of his face, and portions of the right leg. Vera told Audry, the head nurse, "I'm putting down in the chart that he is 20 percent full-thickness burns." Audry concurred, "Yes, that seems about right, although at this point, with that head injury, his burns are the least of the kid's problems." Nevertheless, Sandi, the occupational therapist, appeared shortly after Lonnie was admitted, to measure him for the position splints that all burn patients required.

In the family waiting room, the attending surgeons gave Lonnie's mother a grave prognosis. They informed her that while Lonnie was acutely burned, the head injury was the most life-threatening of his injuries and his chances of recovery were indeed very low.

Much to everyone's great surprise, Lonnie regained consciousness ten days later after being in a deep coma virtually the entire time. As his brain injury began to stabilize, his burns took on new significance, and the burn injury became his major physical problem. Within a few days after Lonnie regained consciousness, he was taken to surgery and had most of his wounds debrided and grafted. Lonnie remained a patient on the burn unit for several months and though there were a number of complications associated with his recovery, eventually he returned home.

We find in Lonnie's case, that the severity of the burn wound was evaluated by staff in relation to his other trauma. Considered apart from his massive head injury, Lonnie's burns were thought to be serious, but his chances of survival would have been considered high. The complications of the brain injury confused the initial prognosis. Trajectory here was difficult to formulate in that no one among the staff knew with certainty whether Lonnie would survive the brain injury, and thus the burn trajectory was clouded. However, in so far as he was admitted to the burn unit, there were attempts by staff to define the future of the burn injury, and his daily wound care was carried out "as if" he were a viable burn patient. While Lonnie was comatose he was primarily a neurological trauma patient and secondarily a burn patient; when he regained consciousness and his neurological condition continued to improve, his burn patient status became primary and within a week or two, his identity as a burn patient on the unit was firmly established.

As part of the Initial-Preparatory Stage, the severity of the burn wound was also evaluated in light of possible complications in recovery, that the staff might have to anticipate. In a temporal sense, each initial trajectory had some element of the future as well as the past. The future had to do with possible complications or problems that might lay ahead in treating the burn wound. No matter how routine the staff might expect a patient's recovery to be, there was usually some voice given to the fact that certain features of the patient's condition was cause for concern. Each patient's initial condition was also considered in light of the past, if not the patient's own medical past, at least, the staff's past experiences with similar patients. Here the initial trajectory might be organized in terms of guarded optimism with respect to recovery; optimistic in that initial assessments of the burn would indicate a routine recovery, but, guarded in the sense that previous experiences with similar patients demonstrated that unforeseen problems could arise. We can see this point more clearly by looking at the case of seventeen month old Lisa James.

Lisa was admitted to he children's burn unit in November, for burns to 45 percent of her body sustained in a housefire. About a third of her burns were full-thickness and included areas of her face, head, forehead, back and hands. Lisa had no significant inhalation injury though she was placed on a ventilator for the first few days. Because of the burns to her face, her eyes were swollen shut and her lips were very thick and puffy. For several days Lisa's head appeared about twice normal size.

Nurses I talked to expected Lisa's recovery to go smoothly as she was a large and healthy baby and did not have a severe inhalation injury. Dr. Mary Eason, the plastic surgery resident, told me, "I think Lisa's got a fifty-fifty chance, but it depends on how quickly she heals. She'll need some grafting done and once we start that it could be a mess. She is burned 45 percent now and with grafts that will increase her burn surface to about 60 percent. Plus, I keep thinking of Andrea right now." I asked Eason, "Who is Andrea?" Eason answered, "She was a little girl we admitted a couple of weeks ago. I guess you must have been gone then. Andrea was burned just like Lisa is. Everything looked routine and then Andrea arrested (cardiac) six hours later. We couldn't save her."

Several of the nurses agreed with Dr. Eason's assessment, while everything about Lisa's condition gave them initial optimism for a routine recovery, their recent experiences of losing a patient who "looked similar" had the nurses leary. As Julie, one of Lisa's nurses explained it, "I'll feel a lot better once we get her fluid resuscitated. That is our major step right now."

During the Initial Stage then, staff were sensitive to the possibility of future complications and problems. Some of these anticipated problems were unavoidable however. Regardless how staff tried to prepare for contingencies and take evasive courses of action, some conditions were inevitable and there was little that staff could do to intervene.

One morning I asked Vera about the situation of Bobby Williams, who was completing his third week of hospitalization for 90 percent body surface burns. "How is Bobby getting along now, Vera?" Vera looked concerned, "He seems to be doing well, but so much of his body is burned there is nowhere to take donor sites. We just can't get him closed, and, of course, the more his wounds are open the greater the chance for infection. We have to wait for his back to heal before he can be grafted again because that is the only place they (surgeons) can take skin from now."

Ten days later, Bobby hit the kind of low point in his recovery trajectory that Vera had feared, Gwenn described Bobby's condition that day for me. "Well, his stomach is all distended now. No one knows why so they're going to take an x-ray. His stomach and bowels have just stopped working. Also his tissue cultures are looking bad; he's infected somewhere. They're (surgeons) going to switch his topical dressings for awhile to see if that will stop the infection. This type of topical that we'll put on his burns has be left open to the air, so Bobby won't be able to leave his room at all. He's going to get more disoriented than he already is! He'll be rough to handle, and I hope we will have enough nurses."

In my interviews with Sheri, she also related to me how complications can confuse the initial trajectories. "You can't always put a lot of faith in a patient's initial physical accomplishments. Patients might be able to be up and walking and then go bad after that. Then they might get septic. We encourage patients to be active throughout their stay to maintain range of motion. But this activity doesn't indicate progress or that they are getting any better. Someone can take a turn for the worse!"

Anticipating complications in the Initial-Preparatory Stage occasionally lead the staff to develop dual trajectories in which death or recovery were equally possible outcomes. During the Initial Stage, there were times in which staff simply weren't sure which outcome was most probable and the trajectory included recovery and death as distinct possibilities. Usually, however, the recovery trajectory was given initial priority until future events proved otherwise or significant enough to produce a trajectory change. For example, with Lisa James, introduced earlier, the staff was cautiously optimistic, although the recent death on the unit was cause for concern. Nonetheless, Lisa was launched on a firm recovery trajectory and the staff expected most things to go smoothly. Jackie Nimms, whose case I want to present now, had an initial trajectory that was much more ambivalent.

Two and a half year old Jackie Nimms was burned severely in a trailor fire when some cleaning materials ignited. Admitted that night to the children's unit, Jackie had 50 percent full and partial-thickness burns to her chin, head, left arm, upper right arm, and extensive areas of her chest. On the night of her admission, surgeons determined that some of her burns were circumferential, and escharotomies were performed: long incisions were made in her burned skin to release the pressure and reduce swelling. Jackie was placed on a ventilator for several days to assist her breathing. Two days following her admission, Dr. Eason took Jackie to surgery and grafted much of her chest and abdomen. While the surgery was uneventful, three days later Jackie's blood cultures were positive, indicating an infection, and she developed a very high fever for several consecutive days.

One week after her admission and four days following her surgery, the staff began showing concern. Only 50 percent of the grafts that were placed on her chest and abdomen took; the remainder fell off. That fact, and laboratory reports on her tissue cultures indicated that Jackie was septic. Kyra, one of the nurses on duty that day, remarked to her colleagues during nursing report, "We've got another Melody Lewis on our hands, don't we?" The other nurses seemed to agree. Melody was a patient, described in Chapter Six, who had died a few months earlier on the unit, after a hospital stay of over forty days. Judy added, "Jackie is just discouraging. She keeps sliding back. Everytime we get her close to moving forward she has a setback. Now she's infected. I don't know why we can't get her going."

Four days after the above conversation, more of Jackie's grafts sloughed off. Paul, one of Jackie's nurses, told me in a discouraged voice, "She is going to be in here for months. None of her grafts are taking and it takes so long to harvest new skin so she can be regrafted." I asked him, "How do you feel she is doing otherwise?" Paul thought for a few moments. "To be honest, I think Helen, Jackie's mom, should be spending more time with her. Jackie could be gone tomorrow. You remember what happened with Melody. She went down in three hours and so could Jackie."

That afternoon in nursing report Paul suggested a line of action for nursing care. He told the other nurses in the room, "We can't give up on her (Jackie). We can't just treat her burns. We've got to give her a lot of social and psychological support. We need to talk to her, tease her and lots of kisses. Tell her we love her. Her dressing changes hurt her like Hell. But you can only say you're sorry so many times. We have to show her we really care."

Thus for several more days, there was confusion in Jackie's trajectory. Her body's rejection of grafts, the continuing infections and other problems, lead the staff to compare her condition with other children who had died. Yet, her age, general health, and other laboratory studies that were encouraging, made a dying trajectory seem somehow inappropriate to the staff. Dr. Eason continued to tell Jackie's mother that she was optimistic about Jackie's recovery chances. Because of the ensuing complications and prediction that Jackie was in for a prolonged hospital stay, the initial trajectory was marked by ambivalency and some degree of vacillation between dying and recovery expectations, although the recovery trajectory was dominant. This was made clear in Paul's comments during nursing report, "We can't give up on her." In effect, Paul was trying to establish a firm and accepted recovery trajectory, despite his own warnings to me a few days earlier that Jackie could go down at any time. Ambivalent trajectories, thus, were difficult for staff to contend with and during the Initial-Preparatory Stage, there was a tendency for staff to attempt to resolve the issue and gain a sense of clarity and more structured expectations. While in the earliest days and weeks of a patient's stay, the number of unknowns about the future course was the greatest, the trajectory allowed the staff to organize their work and understand events in a more structured way. Paul's challenge to the nurses to treat more than Jackie's burns by meeting her social and psychological needs, was based on the assumption of a recovery trajectory, and it was an attempt to reduce ambivalency, and organize and rationalize future recovery work.

The Initial-Preparatory Stage not only marked the beginning of recovery and dying expectations and assessments, it was also a period in which burn unit staff socialized their patients into the role of burn patient. As we learned in preceding chapters, burn victims had little opportunity to prepare themselves for their hospital ordeals. The suddenness and unexpectedness of their accidents, the tremendous physical and mental shock of the burn injury, and their immediate immersion into a critical care setting, left patients frightened, uncertain, disoriented and anxious. Patients were often confused about what had happened to them, how they got to the hospital, and more importantly, unsure about their future as burn patients. During the Initial-Preparatory Stage, staff helped patients come to terms with their anxieties and confusion by socializing them into the role of burn patient, with its clear-cut expectations of behavior, attitudes and values. By learning a role, patients found structure and meaning for their experiences and gained their own sense of trajectory.

The burn unit staff taught patients a number of things about what their experiences would be like and how they were expected to respond to their newly acquired status as a burn patient. Within the first few days, for example, most patients learned not to expect a quick recovery. Vince Musso, a thirty year old male burned on his arms in a gasoline explosion, asked Joan, the physical therapist, on his first day of admission, "Mam, how long am I going to be in here?" Joan was busy adjusting one of his splints as he lay in bed. "I'll let your doctor tell you for sure, Vince, but you better count on several weeks." Vince acted surprised, "Weeks?" Joan nodded, "Yes, Vince. You see these burned spots on your arms?" You're going to need new skin on those areas. This is a special hospital unit to treat people such as yourself who get burned, Vince. Every patient here has been burned and most of them will be here for many weeks. Now I want you to start moving your arm here. We are going to work with your arms every day. Otherwise they will get stiff and you won't be able to move them."

Not all the staff socialization was done directly; often patients learned about their future and what they could expect indirectly as they became learning examples for students. This happened several times, as student nurses and therapists were given instruction in burn wounds through examination of live patients. Patients who participated in these exercises got a glimpse of their situation that they might not otherwise have obtained.

Ron Haynes was twenty-three years old and badly burned in a plastics explosion in his place of work. His face and legs sustained the major injuries and he required extensive surgical grafts. One morning as Sheri was changing Ron's dressings, Maureen entered the room followed by Ginny and Lucy, two student nurses. Maureen was responsible for providing their orientation on the burn unit. Maureen asked Sheri, "Do you mind if we look at Ron, now that you have him open? I want to show these students what fresh grafts look like." Sheri replied, "No, come on in. Ron, do you care if we show these nurses your burns?" Ron shook his head, "It's O.K. with me." Maureen steered the two students to the side of the bed, so they could get a better view of Ron's recently grafted thighs. Sheri told them, "Now these are fresh grafts here above his knee. And you can see they have taken pretty well. See how nice and pink they are? That means they have a good blood supply and that they will probably take." Ginny looked at Sheri and asked, "Will they leave scars?" Maureen answered for Sheri, "Yes, all grafts like that will leave scars. But Ron will be fitted with pressure garments before he is released from the hospital and if he wears them, that will help reduce the scarring. But these are fresh grafts and with time they won't be so discolored. They'll soon lose that pinkish color." Ginny had another question for Sheri, "Will he need more grafts?" Sheri replied, "That's possible. See those areas on the side of his thigh? We're hoping that those spots will heal in on their own, but if they don't, Ron will need that grafted too." Ron laid there in silence, looking at the ceiling as his wounds were discussed. No doubt he was aware of some of the information being relayed to Ginny and Lucy, but, nevertheless, the reality of his situation was all the more reinforced as he heard Sheri discuss his future scarring and need for grafts and as his trajectory was made all the more clear and certain for the students.

During the initial socialization patients also learned to prepare for contingencies in their recovery. Just as the staff tried to prepare themselves for problems in a patient's recovery, so too did patients have to learn that their recovery might not always progress smoothly. Even the length of time involved in the recovery period was something that patients had to adapt to. Although in this matter, the staff rarely conveyed to patients the relatively long time frame that would attend their recovery. Joan Freeman, the physical therapist, told me one afternoon, "Jim, patients often ask me how long they will have to go before they will be back to normal. Well, I just can't tell them that it will be years. At least two years, and more for some patients. So I tell them, 'Let's just get through these first few weeks.' I just don't want them to get discouraged." With staff encouragement patients learned then to break then long rehabilitation process into smaller, and more manageable and better understood periods of time.

Burn unit staff also got patients to realize the full extent and significance of their injuries, particularly in relation to possible disfiguration and residual physical handicaps. Maureen was talking to Britt McCarthy on his second day of admission for severe electrical burns to his arms. As Britt lay quietly in bed with his arms heavily wrapped in gauze dressings, Maureen informed him, "Britt, you have some serious burns and that's why we have you on a heart monitor. Electric burns are a tremendous shock to the heart and we need to monitor you to make sure there was no permanent damage to your heart. Also, Britt, electric burns actually burn from the inside out, and cause severe damage to the tendons and blood supply and nerves. These kind of burns often result in amputation and you might lose your hands. But it is too early to tell right now. We'll know better in a few days."

Phil Richardson, whom we met earlier, was in his third day post-burn, and during his dressing change, Joan was pointing out for me, parts of Phil's wounds that she thought to be third degree. At one point, she poked a section of Phil's skin and asked him, "Does that hurt?" Phil responded, "No, I don't feel it." Joan turned to me, "See?" Phil looked concerned, "Is that a bad sign?" Joan nodded, "It could be, Phil, but we don't know for sure now." Later as Joan was putting Phil through his exercises she complimented him, "Phil, you're as strong as a bull; you'll do just fine in here."

While patients were made aware of contingencies and given guarded prognoses about the potential for future problems or handi-capping, some of the more fortunate were given reason to take heart and have courage. Gary O'Neil, for example, was in his early twen-ties and during his first few days on the unit, he was very anxious and fearful about whether he would fully recover. On his second week, June gave him an encouraging prognosis as a way of stimulat-ing him to take hope. "Gary, look how well your skin is healing. See how easily I can peel off the dead skin here? That's really good, Gary; it shows you've got very good skin." That afternoon I asked June why Gary should be healing so well. June explained, "Well, he's a big strong healthy guy. Those types can respond well to burns. Also, he's not an alcoholic. That's another thing in his favor."

As we learned a bit earlier, patients were taught to think in terms of short periods of accomplishsment and progress, due to the slow, lengthy and complicated process of burn wound recovery. As pa-tients learned that a long road lay ahead of them, they began to look for small progress benchmarks, which were periodic indications that they were indeed moving toward recovery.

The benchmarks took many forms and some of them had to do with the daily laboratory reports and tests that indicated hwo well the patient's physical system was responding to the burn injury. However, as Joel Horling, the plastic surgery resident, experessed it, the daily laboratory reports have to be approached with caution. "These daily lab reports are important, but it takes a bunch of them to add up to a benchmark. It's going to take a couple of weeks to mean something. And for that reason I avoid telling families and patients about the daily lab findings. When we get a benchmark, then I'll tell them. The rest of the time, I want the nurses to keep the families off my back."

Another progress benchmark that patients learned to consider had to do with skin-grafting operations for full-thickness wounds. Assuming that the skin grafts were successful, each operation signaled for the patient that more of her/his wounds were now being closed, and, barring complications, the patient was moving closer to the day when he/she could go home. If the grafts did not take (a process known as sloughing-off), then that indicated a setback in a patient's recovery trajectory and added several more days if not weeks to his/her hospital stay. Many patients hoped their burned skin would heal without the need for surgical grafts and often found that after waiting weeks for their skin to show signs of regeneration, their hopes were in vain. The inevitable surgery that followed was interpreted by patients as a delay in their progress, because of the immobilization that was necessary for several days after surgery.

Progress benchmarks are also located in the physical exercise routines. Occupational and physical therapists measured each patient's range of motion weekly to check for improvement. As patients were able to increase or at least maintain their range of motion as a result of the exercises, they learned to view this as a sign of their successful rehabilitation. Loss of range of motion over a week's time meant that the patient was not exercising vigorously enough, and that more recovery time in the hospital would be needed if the patient was to approach the rehabilitation standard set by the therapy staff.

Turning finally to the last aspect of patient socialization during the Initial-Preparatory Stage, I want to discuss briefly identity change, which was the process in which patients learned to accept their new status on the burn unit. In the earliest days and weeks of their hospitalization, patients had to prepare themselves for a new identity as burned persons with all that was implied in terms of scarring and disfigurement. For many patients, the process meant that a new life had begun, and without fully realizing at first, there was no returning to the former identity and status. Those patients whose burns were to leave them scarred, mutilated, and facially disfigured found that their recovery in the burn unit was more than a passage of time through a recovery trajectory, it was a self-transformation, shedding an old identity for a new one. This transformation process did not occur entirely in the Initial-Preparatory Stage. The process was much more gradual and unfolded throughout a patient's hospital stay, and, for many, extended well into their at-home recovery period. But during the initial socialization, staff began to awaken in patients the possibility that at least some aspects of a new life had begun. The burn team felt it important that patients accept the reality of the burn unit, and their special status within it. While many burn patients wanted to be left alone, or allowed to die, or refused to accept what had happened to them, and in their fears and anxieties wanted to retreat and withdraw psychologically from their plight, the staff would not permit it. The Initial-Preparatory Stage was not a grace period. Whatever patients had to do, or to learn, or to believe in, to promote their recovery was begun within days of their admission. Socialization into the burn unit setting, into the demands of the Program, and into a new identity was now beginning. Whether they liked it or not, patients were pulled, pushed, and prodded, sometimes kicking and screaming into the world of the burned.

Normalizing Stage

This stage fits rather loosely with the time period covered by the Acute Phase of physical recovery. Normalizing was not a fixed period of time, tending to vary with how the staff perceived each patient's needs. In general, however, normalizing accompanied the middle weeks of the recovery trajectory, when staff fully expected patients to live and be rehabilitated from their burn injuries. During this period patients' physical conditions were stabilized, or nearly so, they were usually successfully fluid resuscitated, and some degree of wound healing was taking place. For most patients, the middle of the trajectory saw the removal of urine catheters, heart monitors, intravenous lines and ventilators. As a result, patients were required to spend less time in bed, and were free to visit the television lounge to meet other patients and compare experiences. In this period of time, patients were gradually coming to terms with the burn unit setting, learning its rules, codes of behavior, values and ideals. Everyone in the unit was on a first-name basis, staff and patients alike, and except for consults and personnel from other wards, no one was a stranger. At this point in their recovery, patients were seeing the burn unit for the first time as a social world.

The Normalizing Stage found patients settling into the daily round and routines involved in their care: the morning tankings and dressing changes, physical exercises and the other Program activities described in Chapter Five. As patients now no longer expected or wanted to die, the question for the staff became: how would patients live? That is to say, how would patients endure and live up to all the varied and difficult demands of their recovery? At this point in trajectory, the staff were most concerned with the morale or emotional well-being of their patients. Could patients cope with and accept all that would now be expected of them in their recovery?

One of the ways staff got patients to accept their present situation and future obligations was through the normalizing process. This process was actually part of the rehabilitation plan, to get patients to respond normally to what had happened to them and to instill in patients the idea that they were normal people. Though the burn unit setting was unlike anything patients had ever encountered, staff encouraged patients to view their lives and activities within the setting as predictable and normal. During this stage, staff tried to create a sense of continuity and connectedness for patients between their hospital life as a burn patient and their home and family situations. While many patients had to accept a new identity as a scarred and disfigured person, the staff encouraged patients to see that new identity in light of old identities and familiar statuses. The transformation was to be gradual rather than abrupt and linked with what was known and familiar. In the Normalizing Stage, patients learned to take hope and courage and to respond to challenges in ways considered familiar, normal, and appropriate.

Sheri, during an interview, talked once about patients' emotional recovery from burns, "You want patients to act normally in situations. And this is not easy because patients have so much stress to relate to." I questioned Sheri further, "What happens when patients have trouble handling that stress?" Sheri continued, "Many patients regress. Even though they are adults, they start acting like babies.

They whine and complain, and get demanding and immature. And it's the pain that does it. Constant pain makes them regress. Some patients don't come back to normal until they are ready to go home. I feel that a patient's physical recovery comes before his/her emotional recovery."

As part of the Normalizing Stage, the burn unit staff expected patients to get discouraged about their slow progress, possible setbacks in recovery timetable as well as in their uncertain futures as disfigured persons. If regression was an adaptation to the effects of physical pain, depression was a response to the emotion pain of discouragement and delays in recovery. Sheri, expressed this depression reponse this way, "It's fairly typical for patients to get depressed. Some men get depressed if they don't tolerate pain very well. Later when they are ready to go home, patients get depressed about their physical appearance, because they know people will stare at them. And most often, patients just feel that they should be getting better faster. They don't realize, even though we try to get them to, that recovery from a burn is a long slow process. There are no short-cuts. So we encourage short-term goals. Patients have to look at things from day to day and not worry about a year from now."

During the Normalizing Stage, even the children perceived the long arduous nature of their recovery. Children especially became discouraged with repeated surgeries and the pain and discomfort experienced in the post-operative recovery. Earlier in this chapter we studied the case of seventeen month old Lisa James, who was burned on 45 percent of her body in a housefire. One afternoon I was visiting Lisa, as she was being held and cuddled by her mother, Joyce, and her Aunt Dianne. The previous day Lisa had undergone a fourth skin grafting operation. The surgeons had grafted parts of her face and ears and had sewn a large gauze packing into the side of Lisa's face to hold the grafts in place. As a result, her face now was very puffy and swollen. The three of us tried to get Lisa to smile or react, but to no avail. Though we took turns holding her, Lisa acted indifferent to each of us and her face was fixed with a scowl. Joyce was somewhat hurt and disappointed, "She's mad at me and she won't even look at me. I hope she gets over it. She doesn't like what's happening to her and I guess she blames me. You know, before she got burned she was always in a good mood." As we continued to comfort Lisa, Joyce talked again about Lisa's moods, "It's funny. Lisa doesn't even cry normal anymore. She usually has a loud, piercing cry. But in here (burn unit) it's a dry cry and you can hardly hear her!"

Staff encouraged patients to look for small signs of wound healing in the Normalizing Stage and to take pride in even minor acts of independence. As Sheri pointed out earlier, patients were taught to think in terms of daily accomplishments and small benchmarks of progress. Gradually patients had to accept the idea that there would be no dramatic breakthroughs or abrupt changes in condition. Patients learned also that they could help their rehabilitation by cooperating with staff in the Program.

Gary O'Neil, whom we met before, had 35 percent burns on his arms, shoulder, neck and parts of his face. Having a high pain tolerance, Gary had developed a reputation as a fairly cooperative patient. Consequently his hydrotherapy sessions and dressing changes usually went smoothly and he did little complaining. After one of his morning dressing changes in the tank room, Vickie was putting a hospital gown on him to take him back to his own room. Gary stopped her, "I would really appreciate it if you would go to my room and get me a pair of those scrub pants. I hate these gowns." Vickie agreed and sent me to get Gary a pair of pants. She was willing to do this I think for two reasons. One, taking time to retrieve a pair of scrub pants for Gary was a small reward acknowledging his cooperation during dressing changes. Two, Gary's desire to wear pants was an attempt to normalize his situation on the burn unit, and it was this kind of independence during the Normalizing Stage that staff looked for in patients.

Likewise, staff pointed out small indications of progress as a means of instilling patient motivation, in the face of many discouraging aspects of patient recovery in the Normalizing Stage. As Audry, one of the nurses interviewed, told me, "We point out the skin buds to patients. That's a sign of healing. And we basically tell them, 'I know it hurts, but now you are on the way.' Unfortunately, a lot of patients lose all motivation now. Patients get discouraged when their wounds look gross. We (nurses) will look at a patient's wound and say, 'Doesn't that look good? Look at those skin buds!' And the patients will respond, 'God, that looks awful!' But we have to point out the encouraging signs. However, we don't tell them about the itching. Once they start healing they will itch terribly. But at this point, we only stress the positive."

By persuading patients to see the encouraging aspects of their recovery, staff were actually getting patients to look toward a meaningful future. While patients had to accept their new status as burned persons, and to realize that some residual scarring and handicapping were inevitable, nevertheless, patients were lead to believe that their lives could go on as before. Part of normalizing meant that as patients looked for short-term goals of physical progress, they were at the same time to envision a future for themselves as normal, functioning persons. Thus, the staff continually prodded patients into talking about future marital plans, dating relationships, their children and grandchildren, and their jobs and work careers. Patients were rarely, if ever, told that any of these statuses or relationships would have to be forfeited or curtailed because of the burn injury and its effects. Moreover, patients were never permitted to express self-pity or remorse or to talk as if their future was bleak. While they might not be exactly the person they were before the burn injury in terms of physical appearance and ability, patients were frequently reminded that they could have a post-hospital life that would be meaningful and rewarding.

Ron Haynes' case is worth examining to illustrate the normalizing process. On an October afternoon I was in Ron's room as Sheri was taking time to adjust his position splints. Burned severely on his legs and parts of his face and upper body, Ron had been confined to bed for several days now following skin graft surgery on his right leg. Ron was about a month away from being able to return home. Sheri asked Ron, "Do you think that you'll go back to work at the same place, Ron?" Ron responded slowly and quietly, "I just don't know. After that explosion, I'm beginning to wonder if that plant is such a safe place to work. I wouldn't want to go through this again." Sheri continued her work on the splints, and then paused to ask him, "You're getting married too pretty soon, aren't you?" Ron agreed, "Yes, you know we were supposed to get married this Winter, but I think we might have to put it off for awhile." Sheri nodded, "I see what you mean. But I'm sure that Janice (Ron's fiance) won't mind waiting a little while longer. You've got a long time to get married."

The normalizing process extended not only to giving patients a sense of a future, but also the patient's everyday life on the burn unit. Though their patient status on the unit was primary, the staff saw to it that other normal statuses of the patients did not recede entirely into the background. If patients were to invest themselves in a meaningful future, they had to see some connection between their future and the present situation. Staff accomplished part of this through appearance work, normalizing as much as possible the patient's physical appearance, and also by encouraging activities that would connect patients to the outside world. For example, patients were persuaded to be out of bed during much of the day, to spend time in the lounge watching television with other patients, to have radios in their room, and to receive visitors.

Appearance work was a key element in normalizing, since patients during this period were becoming sensitive about their scarring and disfigurations. While little could be done to make burned skin appear attractive, staff made certain that patients brushed their teeth, combed their hair, and that the men shaved daily. Nurses even searched for after-shave cologne and perfume for patients to improve their attractiveness.

Gary O'Neil was in the hydrotherapy tank one morning and his nurses noticed his fresh hair cut, that one of the evening shift nurses had given him. June teased him, "Why Gary, look at you. You've gotten better looking over night! Does Adele (Gary's wife) like your new hair style?" Gary grinned sheepishly, "I guess so. She said it looked a lot better than before." June continued, "Why yes, I bet she thinks you are pretty cute now."

During visiting hours, I entered Phil Richardson's room and he was sitting up in bed. Earlier that day he had gotten his hair washed, and his nurse had brushed it thoroughly for him, and had put a nice part in it. I remarked, "Phil, you look like a new man. Are you going out tonight or something?" Phil managed a rare smile, "Well, the next best thing. I get to see my young-un tonight. Irene (wife) is bringing him up and the doctors said it was O.K. if I walk down the hall to see him." I asked Phil, "Is this the first time you've seen your son since you were burned?" Phil replied, "Yes, it's been over a month now. I wonder what he'll think when he sees his daddy looking like this? Hope I don't scare him."

Children too were normalized, in fact, the process with them started somewhat earlier than adults. Within the first few days of a child's admission, toys were attached to their beds, balloons hung from IV poles, and even cassette recorders were placed on their beds so that children could listen to songs and nursery rhymes.

After Lisa James had been on the unit nearly three weeks, Dr. Eason, the surgery resident, gave me a progress report. "I'm thinking of taking out her catheter and if she can start taking things by mouth we can discontinue her IV in a few days. Then we can get her up and looking like a little kid again."

A few weeks following that conversation Lisa, who was seventeen months old, was going regularly to physical therapy. The nurses were dressing her in color coordinated children's clothes rather than in hospital garb. Lisa wore a thick net that covered the entire top of her head since all that surface had been grafted, and the nurses pinned bright blue and green ribbons on the net each morning. One afternoon she was returning from physical therapy and riding in the wagon being pulled by the therapist. As she entered the unit she waved "Hi" to everyone and in return several of the nurses standing there told her how cute she looked with her new ribbons.

In the later phases of the normalizing process, a patient's recovery was, in a sense, a social as well as physical state. As patients began to show signs of physical improvement, the burn staff expected them to act in ways that demonstrated a socio-emotional readiness to leave the hosptal. However, as Sheri indicated earlier, there was usually a gap between a patient's improving physical status and his/her emotional recovery or coming terms. At a certain point in the Normalizing Stage patients began to heal and recover relatively quickly compared to earlier phases in the trajectory. While staff and patients alike welcomed this rapid physical improvement, staff were always sensitive to the patients' social and emotional progress and whether patients were fully capable of dealing with the fact that they might soon be going home.

Thus some patients became depressed and discouraged at the very time their physical condition was greatly improving, and their rehabilitation outlook was the brightest. This contradtiction between morale and physical recovery can be illustrated by looking at some of the events surrounding the care of Gary O'Neil, whom we've talked about before.

Gary had been hospitalized for well over a month when his physical status began to change for the better and there was talk among the staff about sending him home in a few weeks. He had an early reputation on the unit as a cooperative patient and one who tolerated pain very well. However, after a month as a patient, he became increasingly sullen and withdrawn. In talking to Betty, the unit social worker, I learned that Gary's wife and family had not visited him much in recent days. Though they saw him frequently when he was first admittd to the unit, now that he was getting better, his family wasn't around as much. Betty continued, "I had a chat with Gary yesterday and he was really depressed. I felt he was about ready to cry. For one thing he's worried about how his face looks. So I tried to reassure him about that. Also he's worried about his finances. He can't work now that he's in the hospital and he knows it's expensive to be on the unit. Everything seems to be bothering him." Vickie, one of the nurses most concered about Gary, told me, "He just seems to have given up. But I guess he needs a lot of TLC (Tender Loving Care) at this point. We have to show that we still care about him. He's so close now to being well!"

Lonnie Gorham's care provides us further insight into this issue. Lonnie was a seventeen year old high school student, burned in a car accident and facially disfigured. One entire side of his face required grafts and he also lost the eye on that side as a result of his injury. As a temporary measure he had been wearing a black eye patch for several weeks. Lonnie had not seen his appearance until six weeks after his admission to the burn unit. However one afternoon I went to his room for my daily visit with him and after several minutes of conversation I noticed he was very quiet and distracted. Pulling a chair close to his bed, I asked him, "Lonnie, is everything O.K.?" Lonnie was on the verge of tears, and shook his head, "I don't think so, Jim." I coaxed him, "What's the matter, Lonnie?" He answered in a whisper, "I found a mirror in the drawer there and I looked at myself. I didn't realize that I looked that bad." After a moment's pause, I asked him, "Have you told anybody that you did that?" Lonnie whispered, "No, you're the first. My God, Jim, I look awful!"

Lonnie was upset by this for some time and the staff brought up his situation in Team Conference. After much discussion, it was decided to call in a mental health consultant to talk to Lonnie. However, even weeks later Lonnie continued to have difficulty coping with his appearance. In one corner of his room Lonnie kept a large, framed color picture of himself in his prom suit, which was taken only days before his accident. Whenever anyone entered his room to visit, Lonnie never failed to ask, "What do you think about the handsome guy in that picture there?"

Despite the emotional difficulties faced by many patients in the Normalizing Stage, some managed to deal fairly well with the emotional dimension of their recovery. As these persons improved physically, their spirits seemed to lift, and their disposition and outlook brightened. Such patients look forward to seeing the end of their ordeal, and realized that however altered their appearance was at the very least they were well enough to go home.

Nearing the end of a three month stay in the burn unit, Bobby Williams, burned over 90 percent of his body, was having his dressings changed one morning and Maureen was encouraging him, "Bobby, your skin is really getting better. Look at how you're healing now. You've still got a ways to go, but you're getting there." Bobby happily agreed, "Yeah, I can see the light at the end of the tunnel. I'm on the backstretch, aren't I? You know, for a long while I looked like something the cat dragged in to scare the mice with!" Maureen laughed, "Yes, and remember when you used to hallucinate all the time? God, Bobby, you always thought there were little kids running around in your room!" Bobby smiled, "That was in my far-out days, Maureen. I didn't know what was going on then."

As mentioned earlier, in the latter phases of the Normalizing Stage, and somewhat prior to the Dispositional Stage that I will discuss momentarily, many patients were anxious to go home and leave the burn unit behind them. For those patients who had made steady recovery progress, setbacks in timetables there had an especially demoralizing impact on them. Most of the setbacks occurred with failures in wound healing, when the staff discovered that surgical grafts would be necessary to close the wound. When patients faced surgery near the end of the recovery trajectory, they invariably got upset and discouraged.

Such was the case with Alan Scott, twenty-four years old and burned in an industrial explosion. Alan had been a patient on the burn unit for over a month and his recovery was uneventful and routine until the week before he expected to go home. Audry was his nurse on the day in question and she was changing his dressings in the shower room. As she unwrapped the donor sites on his legs she looked at the wounds closely, "Alan, I don't want to discouarge you, but your donor sites aren't healing enough to go home." Alan looked at her and responded, "Can't I take care of them at home?" Audry nodded in agreement, "Yes, you can. Can Erica (Alan's wife) help you?" Alan said that she could.

Audry left Alan in the shower and as she walked into the nurses station she informed Sheri, "I think Alan's donor sites have converted to full-thickness. He's got a whole patch on his right thigh. Maybe someone (residents) got carried away in surgery and went too deep on his donors." Standing close by, I asked Audry what would happen. She replied, "He might have to go back to surgery and get those areas covered." Aurdy let out a sigh, "And here we were ready to send him home next week-end." Audry phoned Dr. Anson, the plastic surgery resident, to tell him what she had found. "Dr. Anson? This is Audry. I think Alan's donors have converted to full-thickness." Dr. Anson replied, "Oh, shit!" Audry was grim, "That's my reaction exactly. What are you going to do?" Anson thought a moment, "For right now, wait and see what happens. They might heal in. I'll look at it later today."

The following morning Glenda was Alan's nurse and as she was changing his dressings she told Alan, "Do you know that you're scheduled for surgery tomorrow?" Alan cried out, "On, no! Not me?" Glenda nodded, "They're going to do those spots on your legs. Didn't Anson tell you about it this morning?" Alan was upset, and his voice was tight. "No, he didn't say anything." Glenda, "Well, that's what they are going to do." Alan began to whine, "I don't think I need surgery. It looks O.K. to me." Glenda said in a soft voice, "I know what I would do." Alan prodded her, "What, Glenda?" She continued, "I would wait and see how it heals. It could heal itself up. This is your choice, you know." Alan perked up, "Well, I don't want it. Couldn't I get a second opinion or something?" Glenda asked him, "In other words, you don't want the surgery?" Alan, "Why, no!" Glenda left the shower room and said over her shoulder, "Then I'll call Anson and see what he says." Returning a few minutes later,

Glenda stood in front of Alan to get his attention. "O.K. Here are your options. You can have surgery tomorrow or go home and see how it heals. But it will take awhile and you'll have to learn to change those dressings, but I'll teach you." Alan said brightly, "I want to go. I know I can change those dressings!"

Later that day Dr. Anson appeared in the burn unit and found Alan in the exercise area. He explained to Alan about the importance of good home care and admonished him to keep his clinic appointments. "If it doesn't heal you'll have to come back and we'll lay more skin." Alan nodded and then questioned Anson, "How did this happen to my donors?" Anson looked away, "Well, we went a little deeper on the graft than we had planned to."

Glenda's action on Alan's behalf was not unusual. When patients had fears of surgery, nurses would call the resident in to try and relieve the patients' anxieties. And in Alans's case, where there were options, especially in the later phases of the recovery trajectory, nurses, on occasion, informed the patient. Presented with choices, some patients would opt to return home hoping their wounds would heal with time. And a few of these patients eventually realized they were postponing the inevitable and had to return to the hospital for additional surgery.

Dispositional Stage

We now turn to the final phase of the recovery trajectory which I refer to as the Dispositional Stage, in that this period involves a variety of decisions concerning a patient's readiness or preparedness to return home. This stage includes the patient's final days or weeks on the burn unit, and it is a time when the staff consider a number of medical/physical, social, and emotional factors in deciding to send a patient home to her/his family and community. Actually, these are group decisions arrived at through the exchange of information and ideas among surgeons, nurses, therapists and social workers during Team Conferences and Grand Rounds. The medical director and the surgery residents had the final authority, however, in deciding to release a patient, and, as we shall see later, there were occasional conflicts among staff as to the readiness of certain patients to leave the hospital.

Burn patients moved into the Dispositional Stage with the gradual improvement in their physical condition. Usually this meant that the majority of a patient's wounds had healed, and that she/he was free from infection, and all surgical grafting procedures were completed. In general, patients graduated to this stage only when the surgeons decided that their work on behalf of patients was pretty much finished. While many patients would have to return to the hospital eventually for reconstructive surgery and surgical release of contractures, these procedures were rarely carried out until a patient had been at home for at least several months.

Whereas surgeons tended to move patients into the Dispositional Stage in terms of wound closure and physical healing, nurses and therapists tended to be more sensitive to and concerned about the rehabilitation function. That is, to what degree was a patient fully independent? How capable was a particular patient in carrying out activities of daily living? Since therapists and nurses spend much more time each day with patients than the surgeons, they were more informed about each patients's ability to adapt both physically and socially to life outside the hospital. Consequently, nurses and therapists were reluctant to send patients home whom they felt needed a lot more work in therapy to become physically independent.

This point is illustrated in the case of Grady Swanson, a twenty-three year old factory worker, critically burned in an explosion at work. Grady survived a tremendous blast that killed a co-worker, but sustained burns on 95 percent of his body. As a result of his burns, Grady was left facially disfigured and physically limited. Grady had been a patient on the burn unit for over three months, when Maureen related to me a conversation she had with Dr. Williams, the medical director. "Williams told me this morning after Rounds that once they (surgeons) graft a few more spots on Grady Swanson next week, then they will be finished with him." I asked Maureen, "Do you think they will want to send him home?" Maureen replied, "Well, I hope not, because he's not ready to go home yet. He still needs a lot of therapy before he can go home. He has got to learn to brush his teeth and go to the bathroom by himself. He can't do any of these things now." Maureen paused to reflect for a few moments, and then continued, "And it's not only that. Grady may get very depressed when he gets home and finds out he's not ready. His family isn't prepared either. You've seen how he looks now. Grady's wife is very young and with two small kids. Can she handle all that?"

The Dispositional Stage did not always proceed smoothly as setbacks in recovery progress were possible. Wounds that appeared to be healing could get infected or break down, the final series of grafts might not get a good take and require regrafting, or a patient who had been free of infection for several weeks could become infected shortly after the staff had decided to send her/him home. Those patients looking forward to leaving the burn unit were always prepared cautiously about their release dates. Patients were rarely given a specific date much in advance; they were offered usually a range of time, announced to them in Grand Rounds. "You can probably go home towards the end of next week."

Staff at all levels preferred to hedge on their predictions for patients concerning release dates. They wanted to avoid conflict with patients and their families that would inevitably result if a firm date was given and then not followed through on, if staff decided to keep the patient a few more days. Thus patients were given release dates only as "maybes" or "possiblys" with much cautionary advice about the possibility of setbacks in progress. A few patients never knew with certainty their time had come until the very morning of the day they were to go home.

Dan Howell was a patient on the burn unit for three weeks. In his early forties, he had been burned on his arms in a gasoline explosion. On the day this conversation took place, Dan was hoping to return home the following week. Glenda was Dan's nurse that day and as she was looking carefully at his wounds, she told him, "Some of these areas on your shoulder still look a little moist, Dan. I don't think you're ready to go home yet." Dan answered her, "Dr. Nowicki said I would be ready some time next week." Glenda shook her head, "Well, they (surgeons) have been known to change their minds. Is your wife coming out to visit tomorrow?" Dan replied, "Yes, she'll be here all day tomorrow." Glenda was pleased, "That's good; we'll start showing her how to change your dressings. Do you think she can learn to do that? If we send you home, she'll have to help you." Dan nodded egagerly, "Oh, I know she can learn to do it. She wants to." Glenda, "Well, I just want you to know that you still have some open areas and you can get infected and make it worse. If you go home, you will have to be very careful with those dressings."

Trajectory conflicts among surgeons and nursing and therapy staffs were most likely to occur during the Dispositional Stage. With some frequency, surgeons were willing to send patients home sooner than the therapists and nurses would have liked. Usually these disagreements were negotiated and compromises were reached during Grand Rounds or Team Conference, and in such cases surgeons agreed to keep patients on the unit a few more days enabling the therapists and nurses to complete their work.

On a few occasions, patients were sent home by surgeons against the judgment of other team members. Artie Hogarth's case represented the type of conflict that could occur between surgeons and other staff.

Artie, sixty years old, had been hospitalized for over two months, and the surgery residents were anxious to send him home, but there was one small wound area on his back that was not completely healed. The options were to graft that wound surgically which would keep Artie on the unit for two more weeks, or send him home in the hope that the area would heal on its own in a month's time. The entire burn team assembled in Artie's room on Monday Grand Rounds, and heard Dr. Horling ask Artie, "Well, are you ready to go home, Artie?" Artie was all smiles, "Yes, I'm ready to hit the road." Everyone laughed with him. Sheri, his nurse, reminded him, "Artie, you've been in here the longest of any patient on the unit right now. You're really the old-timer!"

After the team had departed from Artie's room, Dr. Williams addressed the group in the hall. "He's still got a small spot on his back that doesn't look good. We can send him home, but if it doesn't heal, he'll have to come back and have it grafted." Dr. Horling added, "Artie told me that he's afraid of having his house burglarized. He's been away so long." Williams thought for a moment. "Let's do it this way then, Joel. Why don't you talk to Artie later today and explain his alternatives to him. We can graft him now, or he can go home and see if it will heal there." Horling agreed.

Later than evening I visited Artie's room and asked him what he had decided. He was emphatic, "I'm getting out of here. I don't want no more surgery. When I get out of here, I know how to take care of myself. I'll know what to put on it."

Artie was sent home two days later, and on his second day home Artie's wife called the burn unit to report that Artie felt sick and couldn't sleep. Joan Freeman, the physical therapist, told me, "No wonder he's sick. He wasn't ready to go home! He still had that big open area on his back. He could get that infected. Jim, I'll bet Artie's back here on Monday." Betty, the unit social worker, had joined us. "I guess Williams got concerned when Artie told Horling that his house might get robbed. I mean they knew that Artie really wanted to get home." Joan looked puzzled, "Well, that's another thing that doesn't make any sense. Artie never told any of us about those fears. Where did Horling get that? I asked Artie's wife on the phone about it and she didn't know what I was talking about. They've never been robbed and she wasn't afraid to stay in the house. I just don't get it, Betty. On Monday, Williams is talking about grafting Artie and the next day they send him home!"

A similar conflict occurred with Ned Rice, who was thirty-eight years old and hospitalized for seven weeks. After looking at his wounds on Monday Grand Rounds, Horling and Williams decided to send Ned home. In the nurses' lounge that afternoon, Vickie was telling Sheri about her concerns, "I don't think Ned is ready, do you? That area on his shoulder isn't good. I don't think that Williams looked at that graft very closely this morning." Sheri seemed to agree, "It's not only that graft on his shoulder, a lot of grafts have little black spots on them that just look bad." Vera, one of the other nurses added, "They're going to send him home no matter what. They want that bed empty in case they need it." Vickie replied, "Well, Ned will have to come back in before long. That's how I see it."

Despite the occasional disagreements among staff concerning the trajectory and patients' physical readiness to return home, the Dispositional Stage meant, for the entire burn team, that other factors had to be considered in sending patients home. In the last days and weeks of the patient's trajectory, social considerations became as important as the patient's physical/medical condition in making decisions about who could go home. Since most patients were released with some degree for incomplete medical or physical rehabilitation, staff were required to consider the kind of home and family situation the patient would be returning to. For example, upon returning home, patients would usually need daily assistance in changing their dressings, getting their pressure garments on and off, and help and motivation in doing their required exercises. Additionally, those patients with residual physical handicaps, would need a good deal of help in actitivies of daily living, cooking, maintaining their home, and so on. Aside from these considerations, many if not all patients would continue to require much social and emotional support as they made their adjustments to life outside the burn unit. Those patients visibly disfigured would now be trying out new identities and statuses as stigmatized individuals and would need understanding and supportive social networks at home and in their community.

As a result, in making decisions about sending patients home, surgeons always made preliminary inquiries about patients' home and family situations. While the social worker was relied upon for much of this information, surgeons also wanted first-hand assurance when they could obtain it.

During Grand Rounds the team had assembled in Fred Jones's room to discusss the possibility of sending him home. Mr. Jones was in his late fifties and had been on the burn unit for over a month. Dr. Williams stood at the side of Mr. Jones' bed and asked him, "Fred, what about your family? If we send you home, is there anyone there who can change those dressings for you?" Jones replied in a proud voice, "Well, I should think so. One of my daughters is a nurse!" Williams grinned at the other members of the team and then at Mr. Jones. "I could make a smart remark about that, but I fear for my life. Well, how does the middle of this week sound? We'll try to get you out of here then."

On the children's unit, decisions to send patients home depended almost entirely on the staff's faith in the competency of the parents. Children were kept on the unit for longer periods of time if the staff felt that the parents were not emotionally or intellectually capable of giving the child adequate care in the home. In these cases, children were hospitalized until their wounds were healed completely, in contrast to the adults who were sent home often with wounds yet to be healed.

After Monday Rounds, Dr. Coyner was discussing with Kristie, the charge nurse, about which patients, currently on the unit, were closest to being able to go home. Kristie told him, "Susie is pretty

much healed in now. She's still got a few open spots on her arm."
Coyner agreed, "Yes, and her mother seems smart enough to take
care of her. Well, do what you think, Kristie. If you want to, go
ahead and start getting her ready. Maybe by the end of the week?"

Parents on the children's unit were given elaborate instructions
about the at-home care of their children, including at least several
practice sessions in doing dressing changes and tubbing procedures.
Paul, one of the nurses, explained this philosophy, "I like to give
mom instructions for a few days before we send the kids home. It
takes time for all that to sink in with them and it gives enough time
for me to reinforce the important things."

I watched Paul one afternoon with Ruth Peters, whose three year
old son, Mike, had been on the burn unit for three weeks. Paul carefully showed her how to change the child's dressings, how to bathe
him, the use of clean technique and other procedures. Paul also
added, "Now Ruth, don't pamper him either when he gets home.
When kids are up here for along time they try to get away with
things when they get home. Use your normal discipline with him.
Don't let him run the show." Ruth asked Paul, "When do you think
Mike can come home?" Paul answered, "Oh, I think in three or four
days. But don't get mad at me if he's not ready. We don't always
know for sure. O.K.?"

During the final few days of the Dispositional Stage, burn unit
staff not only considered the kind of social and family supports the
patient was returning to, but also, whether the patient was emotionally ready to leave the burn unit. Such emotional readiness
could never be completely gauged, and it did not take priority over
the patients' physical/medical recovery, but it was a factor. Of
course, no staff member could ever know for certain if a patient was
prepared for a life outside the burn unit until he/she left the hospital.
As Audry, one of the nurses, explained to me in an interview, "We
might decide that a patient is physically better, but, we might not
think they are ready to go home. Are they prepared for home, family, and community? Some of our patients tell us that when they
went home, that was their worst part."

Some patients, though badly wanting to go home, nonetheless,
feared that their at-home recovery would not go smoothly and would
require their return to the hospital. This happened a few times

during this research, as burn unit patients learned about the at-home complications of their colleagues who had been released earlier from the hospital. Gwenn told me one morning about her concern for Ned Rice, who had been hospitalized at that point for six weeks. "Ned's worried now that he is going home. He knows that Gary and Phil (patients) who went home a couple of weeks ago are going to have to come back for more surgery. Now he thinks he'll have to come back. I tried to tell him that every case is different, but he's upset about it."

As patients were evaluated in terms of their emotional readiness to leave the burn unit, so too were they gradually prepared to accept the idea that they had to leave. While most patients couldn't wait to get home, there was an ambivalency on the part of many. Though they were anxious to return to their homes, families, and communities, they had grown attached also to many of the burn unit staff and other friends they had made during their stay. For many patients, in the final phase of their recovery, there was a feeling that they had come through some harrowing and trying experience, one in which they had neither fully comprehended nor understood. So that, on the one hand, they wanted to return home and test new identities and statuses, on the other hand, they wanted to come to terms with all that had happened. For weeks and months, the burn unit staff had engaged them socially, emotionally, and physically in the most difficult undertaking of their lives: their recovery from burns. Giving this experience up, as unpleasant and difficult as it might have been, was not easy for some patients.

The staff encouraged patients to break their emotional ties with the burn unit and to rekindle their interests in home, family, and community. For patients who had spent many months on the burn unit, this wasn't easy.

Ollie Wilson was sixty-five years old, and had been hospitalizaed for over four months. Burned severely when he fell asleep while smoking in bed, Ollie had spent nearly a month as a critical-care patient. Nearing the end of his recovery career, Ollie was having his dressings changed one morning by Vera, who reminded him, "Ollie, you might get moved to another ward if a critical patient comes in. You're pretty well healed now." Ollie was annoyed, "Well, I don't want to go. I like it here." Vera persisted, "Ollie, it's you or Sarah

Anderson; you two are the most healed. You've come such a long way, Ollie, do you remember? When they brought you in we didn't think you were going to make it; that's how sick you were then!" Ollie nodded slowly, "I guess I've been through a lot, haven't I?" Vera looked at him, "Oh, Ollie, you sure have. You'll be going home soon. You have got to get ready." Ollie responded, "I don't want to go home. I don't know who will take care of me at home." Vera assured him, "You've got daughters, Ollie; one of them can learn to do your dressing change."

The same week in which Vera talked to Ollie about going home, this case was presented in Team Conference. Virginia, who lead the discussion, informed Dr. Williams, "Ollie's pretty well healed, except for a small part of his back. Do you want to graft it or let it heal on its own?" Williams replied, "Let it heal." Virignia looked around to the rest of the group, "Well, in that case I don't see any reason he can't go home. With such a small area left, he doesn't need to be in here." Williams agreed, "Give him a date so he has time to get ready and he won't think we are trying to sneak up on him."

At the conclusion of Team Conference, Virginia went to Ollie's room and told him of the decision to send him home. Ollie got very upset. Virginia decided not to argue with him, and the next day she sought advice from Betty, the unit social worker. "Betty, Ollie doesn't want to go home. He's so upset he won't eat, exercise, or do anything but lay in bed! Now he says his hip is hurting him!" Betty explained, "Ollie's afraid that no one can take care of him at home. The only one of his daughters that expressed interest in taking care of him is Angie and I suspect that she drinks a lot. I don't kow if it would be good for Ollie to move in with her or not." Virginia was concerned, "Well, he better not burn himself again after all we've been through with him. We didn't think he would make it when he came in. He was burned 55 percent and was such a drinker. But he made it. Now we've got to get him to want to go home!"

Ned Rice was another patient who found it difficult to deal with his emotions about leaving the burn unit. During his final days on the unit he reminded the nurses continuously of how attached he was to them. As Sheri was changing his bed one afternoon, he told her, "I've gotten such wonderful care in this place. I just can't say enough good things about you people. I'm going to miss you all so much, and I really appreciate all you've done for me." Sheri acted somewhat embarrassed at Ned's comments, but smiled at him, "We get a lot of good patients like you, Ned. We get back a lot of satisfaction too."

Before Ned returned home he recorded a message on a cassette for the staff to listen to after he had gone. On the tape he thanked each staff member by name and expressed his deep gratitude. The nurses played the tape on the day following Ned's departure, and several of them were visibly moved by Ned's emotional remarks. I asked Sandi, the occupational therapist, how she felt about Ned's reaction to his experiences on the burn unit. Sandi replied, "You know, Jim, in some ways this place is like Summer camp. Even though you're at camp for only a few weeks, everybody gets so close. I used to cry when I had to leave camp. It was so hard to leave everyone!"

While it would be difficult to imagine how a hospital burn unit could be compared to a Summer camp, Sandi's point contains some sociological sense. The burn unit was for patients a closed setting, an institution set apart, where social relationships were quickly upgraded and made meaningful. Within the space of a few weeks each patient was pulled into a social world that was made to seem real, and, more importantly, they found acceptance as a burned person. During the Dispositional Stage, no patient I observed could look back and say that the experience was pleasant and enjoyable. No one would ever want to relive it. Yet, every patient found some meaning in it, each in his or her own way. Each patient was changed, not only physically, but, also in a social and emotional sense. What was taken from them physically, was gained emotionally by patients in their ability to simply live through the recovery experience. Now at the end of their hospital stay, they stood, as if at the end of a long runway, looking back knowing that they were among those who had lived, and among those whom staff would never allow to give up. Even Ollie Wilson, who didn't want to go home, realized he was a survivor. I'm not arguing here that all patients' experiences were alike, or that they all came to terms emotionally, or that they all went home and returned to normal lives. Many patients did make satisfying at-home adjustments, and some did not. But in their final days on the burn unit, as they tried to sever whatever emotional and social ties they had with the staff and the setting, every patient in their own way knew they had been tested by fire and not found wanting.

Chapter Eight

IMPROVING THE CARE OF THE BURNED:
SOCIOLOGICAL PERSPECTIVES

I THINK it is appropriate to close this book by suggesting some ways that the recovery care of burn patients can be improved. No doubt, the reader has been sensitized already some of these issues that surfaced in the descriptive materials of the preceding chapters. It is necessary, therefore, to make these issues more explicit and concrete by lifting them out of the ethnographic context. However, the suggestion I will make are based on the research findings and the derived theoretical understandings of critical and rehabilitative care. The implications drawn in the pages to follow are not meant to be exhaustive and comprehensive, rather, they are among what I consider the more important concerns that emerged during the research.

Throughout this book I have tried to analyze and understand the care of the burned in terms of the stages or phases that demarcate the recovery career of patients. By means of this phase or stage analysis I sought to uncover and explore the problematic aspects of recovery from burns, both from the point of view of patients and their families, and the hospital staff charged with their care. In keeping with this analysis, I will locate the areas for improving burn care within the three social phases of patient recovery, recognizing that each stage has its own special problems that must be understood within the context of a phase analysis. We will begin our discussion with the Initial-Preparatory Stage.

Initial-Preparatory Stage

Within the initial phase of burn patient recovery, two problem areas can be discerned: one problem has to do with patients' and families' needs for more detailed and structured prognostic information, and the other area refers to the tendencies of the nursing staff to make evaluative judgments about the parents of burned children. Each of these problem areas deserves our closer attention.

Turning to the first issue, I suggest that staff in both the adult and children's burns units give greater recognition to the needs of families and patients for information concerning recovery and dying expectations. In making this suggestion or recommendation, I am fully aware of the very real limitations set by prognostic uncertainty. Recovery from burns as we have seen, is a slow and arduous process, and because of the many sepsis-induced complications that can arise, often it is difficult for staff to give families and patients a clear and precise idea of where a patient stands at any particular moment. The progress benchmarks are indeed somewhat ambiguous, infrequent, and not entirely reliable or the same for each patient. Nevertheless, my research indicates that at almost any point in the recovery and dying trajectories, the staff had a much clearer picture of what was unfolding or about to happen than did patients and families. And unless families were extremely persistent with the staff, such information was not always entirely forthcoming. Moreover, families often receive conflicting and inconsistent trajectory information from different levels of staff. For example, I observed occcasions in which surgery residents told a family member that a patient was doing quite well, and there were reasons for optimism, while the nurses were giving the same family subtle and not-so-subtle hints that the patient's future was bleak. Thus, family members often confided in me that they didn't know who to believe or to turn to for consistent and reliable information.

The more structured family conferences that I described in Chapter Three are an important and necessary vehicle for information exchange between families, and nursing and therapy staffs. When nurses and therapists took the time to formally communicate with families about burn recovery, through the use of films, slides and other didactic techniques, families appeared greatly relieved, and considered themselves better informed. Usually, however, nursing-lead family conferences were given without the input and participation of the surgery residents, who seemed unaware of and even indifferent toward this important information-exchange medium. It appeared that these family conferences were defined solely as a nursing or social work responsibility. This has the effect, it seems to me, of limiting the effectiveness of the family conference. Surgeons have important insights into recovery care, and it is appropriate that their perspectives and information be integrated into the family conference structure. Also, since families looked to the surgeons for authoritative sources of information, their ideas and viewpoints would add weight to what the nurses, therapists and social workers were trying to communicate to families. The family conferences then, should be a team effort, including at various times, the perspectives of all team members, not just the nursing, social work, and therapy staffs.

I further suggest that the weekly Team Conferences, in which representatives of the burn team meet to exchange ideas about the recovery progress of each patient on the burn unit, become a mechanism whereby the prognostic information needs of families and patients are addressed. Team Conferences are the only structured opportunities, aside from Grand Rounds, where the entire team can meet for information exchange and give and take. Since patients and families often received conflicting and confusing information from staff levels, Team Conferences can be used to facilitate communication among team members. It is within this context that trajectory disagreements among staff could be recognized, challenged, and clarified. Though differences of opinion and perspective are healthy and understandable in a team approach to burn recovery and rehabilitation, when these differences remain latent and not subject for discussion, they can only add to family/patient confusion and uncertainty. Though faced with some degree of prognostic uncertainty, the Team Conference should allow staff greater freedom to arrive at more consistent positions and trajectory agreements so that more reliable and certain information is relayed to patients and their families. I want to make clear, however, that in many cases, staff are able to arrive at consistent trajectories and communicate their positions adequately to families. In making the above recommendations, I am referring to primarily those cases where there is significant trajectory differences among staff, which result in confusing messages to families.

Turning to the second problem area of the Initial-Preparatory Stage, we are concerned with the propensity of nurses and other staff on the children's burn unit to make moral and evaluative judgments of the parents of burned children. As we learned in Chapter Three, staff in the children's unit were anxious to involve parents in the recovery care of their children as a means of reducing separation-anxiety, smoothing out the eventual transition for children from hospital to home, and, in general, making the recovery care of children easier to perform. Parental involvement and the twenty-four hour visitation policy lead the burn unit staff to be very sensitive to and concerned about the kind of parents or surrogates with whom they were dealing. One of the ways this concern and sensitivity was expressed was through evaluative judgments about the competency, emotional stability, intelligence, and moral values of the parents.

I would like to point out here, that these evaluative judgments on the part of staff are understandable, when viewed in the context of the burn care setting. During the course of my research, many of the children who were brought to the burn unit were victims of child neglect and abuse. In fact, at one point during the observations, virtually every child on the unit was either a ward of the court, or the subject of police investigation into possible child neglect. Also, there were several occasions when parents readily admitted to being involved in or responsible for the scalding of their own children. The reader can grasp the difficulty faced by the burn unit staff in being objective about or neutral toward parents who stood accused or suspected of child abuse and neglect. Certainly there were pressures in such situations to make judgments about parental competency, ability, and morality. And, it is important to mention, that the nursing staff never made these parents feel unwelcome or unimportant in the recovery care of their children. All parents who demonstrated a willingness to get involved were encouraged by the nursing staff to do so.

Despite this, it seems to me, that in making value judgments about the competency and intelligence of all parents of burned children, the staff ran the risk of creating a self-fulfilling prophecy. That is, to the degree that parents or surrogates are defined as incompetent, unskilled, slow, or irresponsible, they may become so. When the staff expect to get little from the parents, then little is given in return. Within a context of moral and social judgment, it is quite possible that each parent will descend to the lowest level of staff expectation. If there is some truth to this, then these judgments are actually at cross-purposes with the nursing staff's desire to involve parents in recovery care. For instead of bolstering parents' confidence in their ability to participate, the moral judgments can have the opposite effect.

Furthermore, there is a negative effect in all such labeling processes. Once labels are affixed to a person's character, competence, or values, it becomes exceedingly difficult for that person to be seen in any other light. All subsequent behaviors and actions of the person are interpreted solely in terms of the label and not in the context of her/his adaptive responses to particular situations. Thus, I maintain that by making value and moral judgments of parents, the staff are precluding more effective exchanges between themselves and parents. While the staff want to encourage effective parental involvement in recovery care, value judgments and labeling are prohibitive rather than helpful to that end.

I suggest therefore, that in so far as it is possible, these evaluations on the part of staff be held in abeyance. If such judgments are ultimately unavoidable, they should surface later in the patient trajectory, and not at the beginning as the basis of all subsequent interactions between staff and parents. As on the adult unit, Team Conferences take on a special importance in this regard. Team Conferences on the children's unit were often the context or setting in which these early parental judgments were formulated. Burn unit staff spent considerable time in Conference not only discussing the medical/physical conditions of newly admitted children, but, also in making judgments about the competency, intelligence, and other attributes of the parents. Changes in this evaluation process might very well begin with changes in the structure of Team Conferences. While Team Conferences are important for information exchange among staff, they should not be the arena for reinforcing each other's moral and value judgments. Labels and value judgments arrived at during Team Conferences take on a legitimacy and reality they might not otherwise have. This legitimacy dimension makes the labels and judgments difficult for other staff to reject or ignore. Thus, ideas and values promulgated in Team Conference have a taken-for-granted reality to them that all staff feel compelled to adopt.

Perhaps then, by agreeing to eliminate or to curtail judgmental discussion during Team Conference, staff might be better able to postpone judgments, or to individualize them, rather than making them legitimate collective agreements. While the judgmental process may be unavoidable in working with children and parents, by announcing Team Conference off-limits for such discussions, at least the judgments will lose some of their legitimacy and forcefulness, as staff members feel more free to be objective, or hold their own judgments in abeyance.

Normalizing Stage

Looking now at the Normalizing Stage of patient recovery, I should again like to focus on two major issues or concerns that arose out of the research findings: the problematic aspects of helping patients adjust to theirnew status on the burn unit; and the moral dimensions involved in pain management. Let's begin with the adjustment problem first.

I argued in earlier chapters that the Normalizing Stage brought patients some severe adjustment problems as burned persons. It was at this point in their hospital career that patients realized they were seriously injured and their recovery would be slow, complicated and above all, painful. Moreover, at this juncture, the greatest demands were placed upon them in terms of their compliance with the recovery program. As we have seen, patients were required to gain some level of physical independence, endure their pain, exercise daily, and meet their calorie requirements. And equally, if not more important, patients had to begin to accept their identity as a burned person, one who would be to some degree forever scarred and disfigured. In other words, they were faced with the problem of managing a spoiled identity. All of this meant that most patients faced a serious adjustment problem during their recovery in the Normalizing Stage.

While burn unit staff recognized that there was indeed a socioemotional component in recovery from burns, patient adjustment problems were the least understood, anticipated, and even provided for. Whereas patients' every medical and physical problem was probed, evaluated, studied, and meticuously examined, only patients' most obvious and gross behavioral maladjustments were attended to. In effect, and there is much evidence to show that this is true of most hospital recovery programs; patients' medical/physical needs were considered primary, and their socio-emotional problems were viewed as secondary.

This is not to say that the burn units in this research did not make use of staff social workers and mental health consultants, for as we learned earlier, they certainly did. What I'm arguing here, is that in the Normalizing Stage and also in the Dispositional Stage, the difficulties faced by patients in making satisfactory social and emotional adjustments to their status as burned persons was much more profound and complex than most of the staff realized.

The healing process in burn recovery is as much social-psychological as it is physical and medical. Yet, while the staff had a vast and sophisticated technology to assess a patient's physical recovery, e.g., laboratory studies, tissue cultures, etc., their capacity to gauge a patient's socio-emotional recovey from burns was very limited and rudimentary. Each staff member was sensitive to differing emotional needs of patients, and most of the staff tried to help patients come to terms when they recognized a problem, or felt that a patient needed special attention. But such helping efforts tended to be random, and were never systematized, organized, fully planned or integrated with the patient's total needs and concerns. Though each patient's physical progress was carefully charted and recorded, patients' emotional progress was accounted for only in the most general and obvious ways.

To be more specific, on the adult unit, the social worker was charged with meeting and understanding most patients' adjustment needs, but, as her responsibilities extended into many other areas, e.g., helping families secure housing, arranging financial assistance, etc., it was a difficult task at best to anticipate and closely monitor each patient's socio-emotional progress. What typically proved to be the case was that only those patients whose attitudes and behaviors clearly stood out as problematic and disturbing were systematically attended to. Usually, only those patients whose actions disrupted the ward order and began to interfere with the smooth flow of work, were referred for psychological or social work consultation. To paraphrase a time-worn adage here, "The squeaky wheel got the grease!" Conversely, those patients who were quiet, passive, and compliant, were often thought to be making satisfactory emotional adjustments simply because none of their behaviors or attitudes were considered disturbing. As a result, on the adult burn unit, the efforts of the social worker, and outside psychological consultants, usually centered on the most obvious patient problems and those that the rest of the staff felt most disturbing to ward order and routines. To cite an example in this regard, if a particular patient became so depressed that he/she refused to eat, then the social worker, or psychological consultant would be asked to help.

In light of these considerations, I suggest that in addition to the burn unit social worker, there is a need for a fuller integration of social and psychological support services for burn patients. Such support services should not be seen as secondary, or even consultative in nature. Psychological services should be an integral part of the burn care team, not acting on the basis of referrals, but, in terms of serving patient needs in a continuous and comprehensive fashion. Patient adjustment problems during the Normalizing Stage should be anticipated rather than reacted to. Social-psychological care plans for patients are every bit as important as nursing, therapy, and medical/surgical plans, and this idea requires explicit recognition. Just as there are predictable stages of physical recovery from burns, so are there fairly predictable phases of a patient's socio-emotional recovery, and the attending adjustment problems need integrated, comprehensive and continuous support services.

Focusing now on the second problem area in the Normalizing Stage, I would like to say some things about pain management and control. In preceding chapters, I tried to show that during the Normalizing Stage, patients faced their most significant ordeal with respect to pain. Virtually every aspect of their daily recovery care was painful and many patients built up substantial pain-related anxieties. We examined in Chapter Four, the various strategies employed by staff in structuring the pain experiences of patients. Each of these strategies was designed to help patients come to terms with their pain in ways that allowed work routines on the burn unit to proceed smoothly.

I pointed out also in that chapter that while a variety of oral pain medications were prescribed for patients, morphine use was restricted because of nursing staff fears of patient addiction. Moreover, it was felt by the staff that dosages of morphine sufficient to block burn pain would render patients incapable of being actively involved in their recovery. Interestingly, examples from the research literature show that philosophies about morphine usage vary in burn units around the country. Studies on pain control reveal that some burn units use relatively large amounts of morphine in controlling patient pain, some units use hardly any, and other units fall somewhere in the middle, prescribing relatively moderate amounts. There appears to be no uniform or standard approach to morphine usage among American burn units, and little agreement as to what dosage levels are the most effective and safe.

In light of what we know to be the case in burn units generally, and on the basis of my research on a single burn center, we can argue that the area of pain management and control remains ambiguous, vague, and not well understood. My data reveal that while staff are sensitive to the pain experiences of burn patients, there is no systematic way in which the more effective pain-relieving drugs, e.g. morphine, are used. The social-psychological methods of dealing with pain, such as neutralizing the pain environment, are partly effective, and need to be blended with a better understanding of and more systematic structure for the use of pain-relieving drugs.

I'm led to suggest here that burn unit staff be more accountable in managing pain. This same suggestion was made a number of years ago by Glaser and Strauss in their studies of pain control, and it certainly bears repeating today. In many other aspects of patient care, medical and nursing staffs are held strictly accountable for decisions made on a patient's behalf. Yet, in the area of pain control, there is an almost ad hoc, or trial and error approach, in which neither level of staff accepts responsibility or accountability. Pain management practices tend to be seen as secondary to the primary efforts of the staff, attending to the patient's physical/medical recovery. Just as there are no systematic nursing or medical plans to deal with patients' socio-emotional adjustments, so is there lacking definitive plans for pain management. When surgeons write orders for morphine dosages to be given "as needed" and nurses decide to administer those dosages on the basis of their own perceptions of a patient's pain level, this is not an accountable system.

Furthermore, staff reluctance to use morphine at dressing changes or during other painful procedures has a moral dimension to it and patients should be allowed to participate in that decision-making process. Under the present structure the nurses find themselves making such moral/ethical choices, with few structural or organizational guides, other than their own personal beliefs and values. This is a heavy burden of responsibility for nurses to carry, and it should ot be their sole responsibility in the first place. Burn patients should have more optims in pain medications and greater freedom in making moral choices. Whether or not morphine use in managing burn pain can actually result in patient addiction is only part of the issue. What has to be addressed in this regard, is that patients have a right to decide whether they might be willing to take that risk. This is what I mean by the moral dimension in pain management. These are considerations that cannot be decided solely according to staff's morality and values. When pain management practices go beyond strictly medical or nursing judgment, then patients must be given the opportunity to participate in those decisions.

In addition to the above, I also suggest that there is a need to increase the availability of non-pharmaceutical pain relief techniques, such as hypnosis, relaxation therapy, and bio-feedback, as a means of extending a patient's options in pain management. These techniques are being used with some success at a number of American burn centers, particularly at a few of the noted children's burn units. Such efforts at non-pharmaceutical techniques are worthy of emulation. At the burn center which was the focus of my research, these measures were tried periodically with certain patients and were found to be successful under varying conditions. However, techniques such as hypnosis and relaxation therapy were not systematically employed or studied, and they had an ad hoc character to them. In some cases, for example, hypnosis was tried only when a patient requested it, or when all other measures seemed to fail. Likewise, their employment depended on the availability of a trained therapist, and in the absence of such, these options were nonexistent. Thus I recommend that these techniques be made increasingly available to patients, through the hiring of trained staff attached to the burn unit. This would permit a more systematic and organizationally structured use of non-pharmaceutical measures, and their effectiveness could be thoroughly monitored and evaluated. Also, this approach would extend the range of options available to patients which is a key consideration, it seems to me, in pain management.

Dispositional Stage

I described in Chapter Seven how the Dispositional Stage presented burn patients with the difficult challenge of dealing with their at-home recovery. It was at this point that patients faced leaving the secure and accepting environment of the burn unit, where "it was O.K. to be burned." Now they were challenged to return home, to coninue their rehabilitation program, and to try out their new statuses as scarred and disfigured persons. As a number of patients have told me, and as we can learn from reading the published biographies of burn victims, "going home" was really only the beginning of a person's recovery from burns. While many patients thought their ordeal was over, the return home signaled the start of a most difficult recovery period. For no matter how well patients thought they were prepared to continue their at-home recovery upon leaving the hospital, the transition from one environment to another proved especially troublesome.

The transition problems faced by patients were many and varied. Some patients, for example, found great difficulty dealing with the pain and itching that accompanied the continued healing of their burned skin. The pain relief measures that proved somewhat successful for patients in the burn unit often seemed not to work as well in their own home. Other patients were anxious about the ability of their family members to give the quality of daily physical care that they were accustomed to receiving from the hospital nurses and therapists. Dressing changes, for example, that went smoothly and expertly in the burn unit, often were confused and awkward when performed in the home, and patients' anxieties and sense of physical discomfort increased. Still other patients found that the motivational supports they relied on in the hospital to keep them exercising and using their position splints, were lacking in their own home, as family members proved too lenient and sympathetic to push them to their physical limits. As a result, patients began to fear the development of contractures and other deformities as they saw their at-home exercise program gradually abandoned.

Finally, and perhaps most importantly, many patients realized that the identity change they were undergoing was much more trying and perplexing than they had ever imagined. Whereas in the burn center, patients found that most everyone accepted their scars, disfigurations, and altered appearance. Now, in the outside world, patients were being stared at in public, ignored by friends, or worse yet, pitied and felt sorry for by their family. The former secure and familiar reality of their home, neighborhood, and community was now awkward, strange, and uncomfortable. For a few patients, the home they longed to return to was now their prison, and though there were no locked doors or bars on the windows, they did not really feel free to leave. As these patients came to realize, leaving their home meant facing a world where the burned are stared at, pointed to, whispered about, and in other ways made to feel different, ashamed, and no longer normal. The full implications of a spoiled physical identity were now manifest for a number of patients.

On the basis of my research into the world of burn care, several steps can be taken I think to help patients in their at-home recovery, and I would like to suggest some of them now.

To begin, greater attention can be given to smoothing out the transition patients must make from hospital to home. Often this transition is so abrupt, that patients experience the same sense of dislocation they had when brought to the burn unit months earlier. Some American burn units have a step-down structure of rehabilitation in which as patients progress physically they actually move to other hospital wards and units for specialized care. To me, this is an advantageous program as it allows patients to gradually give up the security of the burn unit setting and thus are better prepared to make the transition to home and community.

More importantly, since patients are returning to their families who will become the significant others in terms of socio-emotional support, it is important to get families involved earlier in the recovery care of adult patients. While families were taught how to do the dressing changes that the patient would need at home, such instruction often took place only a day or two before the patient was to be released. It can be argued that if families are to have confidence in their ability help patients in the home, and in turn, the patient is to have confidence in her/his family, such instruction and familiarization should begin earlier. Also, earlier involvement would allow families to become desensitized to the unattractiveness of the patient's wounds, rather than being confronted shortly before the patient is to go home.

Instituting a more liberalized visitation policy on the adult unit would go a long way in accomplishing early family involvement. And, I understand from recent communication I have had with staff at the burn center that this is now being tried and with some success. It was my impression as I visited other burn units around the country that visitation policies tend to be rather restricted. Families were allowed to visit patients only during a few hours per day and at specified times. I suggest that burn centers, for children and adults, place far fewer restrictions on families. (The children's burn unit described in this book can serve as a model.) Patients need the continued and uninterrupted socio-emotional support that their families can give, and families need to be more aware of what patients are going through physically, emotionally, and socially. The kind of awkwardness that patients and families feel toward each other when patients return home is not only unnecessary, but, dysfunctional in helping patients make a satisfying at-home recovery. Much of this awkwardness and lack of mutual confidence can be eliminated by giving families a greater role to play during the hospital recovery, and less restrictive visitation policies.

Another point I would like to make in this regard has to do with the use of home-care nurses especially trained in burn care. I know this program is employed in several burn units in the United States, and I think all burn care facilities should adopt it. No doubt there are a number of geographic and coordination problems inherent in this kind of program and each burn unit would have to take an approach modified to its particular needs and circumstances. Nevertheless, such home-care nursing programs are valuable in giving both patients and families increased confidence in the at-home recovery phase. Furthermore, nurses trained in burn care will be

much more sensitized to patients' recovery needs, even in the socio-
emotional dimension, and can anticipate problems before they become terribly disruptive and difficult for families to deal with. Also,
this program could enhance the continuity of communication between patients and the burn unit, thus improving follow-up care.

Helping patients come to terms with their new identities as disfigured persons is a major problem, and there are no easy solutions
given the nature of society and people's reactions to visible stigma.
However, we know that patient self-help support groups are flour-
ishing and proving successful in helping persons with other types of
disabilities and handicaps, and there is no reason to believe that such
groups would not help the burned. There are national and regional
support groups for burn victims, and it seems that the burn center
has a role to play in seeing that patients are familiar with these or-
ganizations and can gain access to them. Too often, this is defined as
a patient's responsibility, and if he or she does not take the initiative,
nothing is accomplished in this regard. If we can argue that emotional and psychological healing from burns is just as important as
physical healing, then it follows that the burn unit has to assume
greater responsibility in seeing that patients receive adequate socio-
emotional support services during their at-home recovery. Since
these self-help support groups have a good track record in enabling
patients to come to terms, then burn centers need to work more
directly with them in making certain that their patients can become
part of such a program when they are released from the hospital.
Most people would agree, I think, that it does little good to ensure a
person's physical recovery from burns if she or he is not reintegrated
back into society. While not all patients will need this kind of support
group, those that do should not be left to their own devices.

Finally a few words remain to be said about clinic visits. The
burn center that I have described here, and most, if not all, other
burn centers and units in the United States require patients to return to the hospital for period clinic visits. During these clinic days,
as they are usually referred to, surgeons and therapists assess each
patient's physical progress, make decisions about future surgery
needs, and correct problems that have surfaced in the patient's at-
home recovery. Burn unit social workers also play a somewhat active
role in talking to patients and their families about the socio-

emotional adjustments being made in a life now lived outside the burn unit. While it would appear that all the patient's needs are being attended to, I strongly suspect that far less is known actually about a patient's total adaptation to the outside world, than is revealed in clinic visits. For again, it appeared to me that clinic was defined largely as an opportunity to evaluate and monitor the patient's medical/physical recovery. Whatever socio-emotional problems the patient might be having was considered mostly secondary, and seen as the social worker's responsibility. The social workers I observed were certainly well-meaning, anxious to be of help, and professional in their approach, but somewhat inundated by all they had to do for and with patients in the space of a short clinic visit. With many patients to talk to, and many of their needs to address, I wonder how carfully and closely the social workers were able to assess and discover each patient's adjustment difficulties. My observations were that social workers rarely got beyond surface impressions of patients' adjustment problems and thus, dealt primarily with only the most pressing patient concerns. For example, patients might reveal to the social worker that they lost their job, or were forced to find new living arrangements, or similar concerns. Of course these were serious problems for patients and they readily sought and appreciated whatever help the social worker could give them. But in the total context of their social-psychological adjustment to the outside world, these were not the sum total of their concerns or dilemmas. In terms of the whole patient and with respect to the complexity of their adjustment needs, who among the burn team is or should be responsible? While maybe it is too much to expect that in the context of a series of clinic visits the totality of a patient's needs can be examined and assessed, it does seem to be a goal worthy of striving for. Moreover, it appears too much to ask of a social work staff to determine and solve all aspects of a patient's at-home recovery problems that are not specifically physical or medical. There should be a place within the clinic structure for a coordinated effort to meet the needs of the whole patient. The same careful attention to detail that characterized the physical examination must carry over into the social-psychological domain, and all members of the team should recognize this and contribute to that end. If clinic days are opportunities for patients to be "seen," then that vision must not be occluded and concentrated so heavily on the medical/physical plane. Burn patients must be viewed in their totality of being, regardless of the space and time limitations of the clinic setting.

A Concluding Note

Somehow it seems fitting here to add a few brief remarks about my experiences as a sociologist among the burned. Every social ethnographer finds her/himself affected in different ways as a result of being an intimate part of a group or setting over a long period of time. Some of these affects are recognized and acknowledged, while others, I suspect, go unperceived. What becomes affected is not only our professional and academic lives, as we defend and uphold what we have written, but, also, our personal selves, values, and outlooks. It is to this latter aspect that I now want to speak.

For over two years I spent a good amount of my time and energy observing the socio-cultural world of a hospital burn center. Several times during that period a number of friends and associates, who were aware of my research activities, had occasion to ask me, "How can you do that? Isn't it awful seeing people who are burned like that?" To such questions I rarely had an adequate answer, other than to assure them that somehow I had gotten used to it. But, perhaps there is more to it than that, and here is a point worth considering. As sociologists we go where our professional and even personal curiosity takes us. A hospital burn unit is no more difficult or challenging than an urban ·streetcorner, a cocktail lounge, or any other setting studied by social ethnographers. Every setting in which we seek to discover and explain the social arrangements whereby people live, move and have their being, is worthy of study, and all settings are marked by their own special difficulties and liabilities for the observer.

In response to the question, "Isn't it awful?" I could have also said, "Yes, it certainly is." But, what affected me most deeply and personally was not what I saw patients endure while recovering from burns. As the reader must have gathered by now, I observed many dismaying injuries, and witnessed much human suffering and agony. However, the greater tragedy for me was not what patients had to undergo in the burn unit, but the social forces that lead them to be burned in the first place. While many patients in this study were burned through their own carelessness, negligence, or unavoidable accidents, too many of them were injured due to the unsafe working conditions of foundries and factories and as by-products of their poverty. This was especially true of children, many of whom were burned because their houses were inadequately wired, or heated with faulty furnaces, or in other ways unsafe. Such are the housing conditions of low-income people in our society. Likewise, a number of children were burned as a result of parental neglect, which I maintain is also a by-product of adult frustrations with and reactions to a life in poverty and material want.

Social and economic forces lead too many children and working-class adults in our society to be unnecessarily burned. And all the medical technology, which is vast, and all the expertise of surgeons, nurses, and therapists, which is considerable, can ever completely repair the physical and emotional damage caused by a critical burn. While the burned can adapt, adjust and recover, they are never quite the same. When we speak of some people as burn victims, we must recognize that for the impoverished, their victimization started long before they were burned.

One final remark is in order. My reactions and comments above are not meant to deprecate the valuable and skilled work performed on behalf of the burned by surgeons, nurses and other burn care specialists. Nor do I mean to sell short the considerable human good derived from burn care technology. It is always a paradox in American society that our health care technology and medical professionals are asked to do the most for whom the economy has rewarded the least. If we are to have a just and fair society, it seems to me, that we have to address that paradox. And as I think back to the children who were participants in this research, we especially owe this to "the least of these."

BIBLIOGRAPHY

Andreasen, N.J.C., Noyes, Russell., Hartford, C.E., Brodland, Gene., Proctor Shirlee.: Management of emotional problems in seriousnly burned adults. *New England Journal of Medicine, 286, 65,* 1972.
A study of adult burn patients and their reations to current treatment methods. This study stresses the physician's role in relieving patient stress.

Fagerhaugh, Shizuko, Y.: Pain expression and control on a burn unit. *Nursing Outlook, 22, 645,* 1974.
An early sociological study of pain control on a burn unit, that focuses on staff attitudes toward pain and its management.

Glaser, Barney and Anselm Strauss.: *Time for Dying.* Chicago: Aldine, 1968.
This is one of the first studies of hospital death and dying. These authors pioneered the useof the trajctory concept in analyzing hospital work.

Goffman, Erving.: *Asylums.* New York: Anchor Boks, 1961.
Focusing on the career of the mental patient, and the work of psychiatric staff, the world of the mental hospital is examined.

Hamburg, David A., Hamburg, Beatrix., de Goza, Sydney.: Adaptive problems and mechanisms in severely burned patients. *Psychiatry, 16, 1,* 1953.
Using a psychiatric approach, the adjustment problems of burned patients is discussed.

Heidrich, George., Perry, Samuel., Amand, Robert.: Nursing staff attitudes about burn pain. *Journal of Burn Care Rehabilitation, 2, 259,* 1981.
This research is based on a survey of nursing attitudes about burn pain. The authors conclude that nurses do not have adequate knowledge of the pharmacology of pain medications.

Knudson-Cooper, Mary W.: Adjustment to visible stigma: the case of the severely burned. *Social Science and Medicine, 15, 31,* 1981.
A survey research study of the post-hospital adjustments of burn patients. This study indicates that positive adjustments are possible for the severely burned.

Long, Robert., Cope, Oliver.: Emotional problems of burned children. *New England Journal of Medicine, 264, 1121,* 1961

This study maintains that many behaviors of burned children are due to the threat of trauma and enforced hospitalization.

Millman, Marcia.: *The Unkindest Cut.* New York: Morrow, 1976.

A participant-observer study of surgery and its relations to medical control.

Perry, Samual., Heidrich, George., Ramos, Elizabeth.: Assessment of pain by burn patients. *Journal of Burn Care Rehabilitation, 2, 322,* 1981.

The authors report on a survey of the pain experiences of 52 patients. This study concludes that the degree of patient pain during procedures was not related to kind or dosage amounts of pain medication.

Quinby, Susan, Bernstein, Norman R.: Identity problems and the adaptation of nurses to severely burned children. *American Journal of Psychiatry, 128, 90,* 1971.

This research conducted in a children's burn unit focuses on the identity problems faced by nurses in their role as pain-inflicters.

Roth, Julius.: *Timetables.* Indianapolis: Bobbs-Merrill, 1963.

A sociological study of time-passage and patient careers in a tuberculosis hospital.

Solnit, Albert J., Priel, Beatrice.: Psychological reactions to facial and hand burns in men. *Psychoanalytic Study of the Child, 30, 549,* 1975.

This is a psychoanalytic study of the reactions to stigma in young, burned men. The authors stress the importance of meeting the mental health needs of burn patients.

Strauss, Anselm., Fagerhaugh, Shizuko, Y., Glaser, Barney.: Pain: an organizational-work-interactional perspective. *Nursing Outlook, 22, 560,* 1974.

A sociological study examining organizational and work factors in pain control on a burn unit. The idea of pain trajectories is conceptualized in this article.

Ton, Mary Ellen.: *The Flames Shall Not Consume You.* Elgin: David C. Cook, 1982.

This is one of the best written and most revealing first-person accounts of the life experiences of a burn victim.

Weinberg, Nancy., Miller, Norma Jo.: Burn care: a social work perspective. *Health and Social Work, 8, 97,* 1983.

The authors present an overview of social work and the contributions this discipline makes to burn care.

INDEX

259